" 'Culture is not your friend' once said Terence McKenna. The day-to-day life we deem 'normal' involves a form of unseen physical specialization where our movement behavior consists mostly of sitting and walking a few steps, a predicament I have coined as 'movement poverty.' With his brilliant book, Aaron provides us with a stimulating perspective and a simple yet effective method to get us back into better motion, health, vitality and physical freedom."
—Erwan Le Corre, founder of MovNat and author of *The Practice of Natural Movement*

"The first time I met Aaron he was shirtless and barefoot doing a one arm handstand along with some capoeira moves at Onnit Gym in Austin, Texas. Ever since, he has never failed to amaze me, not just with his movement practice, but also with his dedication to helping others reach their full potential. With this book he becomes your personal coach, and you couldn't hope for a better one."
—Jamie Wheal, executive director of the Flow Genome Project

"This is a fabulous book. I don't know anything quite like it. All systems in the body require movement for optimum health. Competent movement that is neither too much or too little, and of the right type is the key. Aaron Alexander masterfully weaves together a formula for successful pain-free living."
—Professor Stuart McGill, author of *Back Mechanic*

"In order to move well, you must move through your own body, investigating its bits, pieces, and perceptions. Aaron masterfully helps you find the keys to your own body home so that you can arrange the furniture of your structure and enlarge your sensual experience of being "at home" in yourself. His book includes wit and wisdom about our sedentariness crisis and easy steps that every human can take to coax their body to be a better citizen within movement culture."
—Jill Miller, author of *The Roll Model: A Step-by-Step Guide to Erase Pain, Improve Mobility and Live Better in Your Body*

"Improving your health and well-being can seem daunting, but really it's a matter of making better decisions on a moment-to-moment basis rather than drastic changes. If you let Aaron guide you as he has me, you'll have the tools to dramatically boost not just your brain health but the quality of your whole life."
—Jim Kwik, CEO of Kwik Learning

"Movement is an important part of achieving high-level wellness that is frequently neglected. *The Align Method* is a wonderful compilation of suggestions to help your body work for you rather than against you. A valuable resource to help you attain the body you have always wanted."
—Dr. Joseph Mercola, founder of Mercola.com, most visited natural health site

THE ALIGN METHOD

5 Movement Principles
for a Stronger Body,
Sharper Mind,
and Stress-Proof Life

AARON ALEXANDER

Foreword by Dr. Kelly Starrett

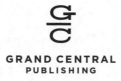

GRAND CENTRAL
PUBLISHING

NEW YORK   BOSTON

Copyright © 2019 by Aaron Alexander, CR, LMT
Cover design by Stef Mcbride. Cover photo by Jeff Skeirik. Cover copyright © 2019 by Hachette Book Group, Inc.

Grand Central Publishing
Hachette Book Group
1290 Avenue of the Americas, New York, NY 10104
grandcentralpublishing.com
twitter.com/grandcentralpub

First Hardcover Edition: December 2019

Grand Central Publishing is a division of Hachette Book Group, Inc. The Grand Central Publishing name and logo is a trademark of Hachette Book Group, Inc.

The publisher is not responsible for websites (or their content) that are not owned by the publisher.

The Hachette Speakers Bureau provides a wide range of authors for speaking events. To find out more, go to www.hachettespeakersbureau.com or call (866) 376-6591.

Library of Congress Control Number: 2019948126

ISBNs: 978-1-5387-1614-4 (hardcover), 978-1-5387-1615-1 (ebook)

Printed in the United States of America

LSC-C

10 9 8 7 6 5 4 3 2 1

"Without deviation from the norm, progress is not possible."

—*Frank Zappa*

Acknowledgments

This book was made possible by the amazing support group around it, including Phil White's countless hours of research, editing, co-writing, and cheerleading. I'm also indebted to my agents, Jaidree Braddix and Celeste Fine, for believing in this project from the beginning. My editor Leah Miller continually refined the message in each and every paragraph, and Kelly Starrett was kind enough to lend his wisdom to the foreword. A big thank you goes to Michael Breus, Patrick McKeown, Wednesday Martin, Ryan Glatt, Jill Miller, Brian Mackenzie, and several others who generously reviewed the content and gave helpful feedback. Finally, I'd like to dedicate this book to my parents, for instilling in me that life is a gift.

Contents

Contents

PART IV. MOVING YOUR SENSES

Foreword

If you pinned me down and asked me upon pain of humiliation and death what I'm good at—like actually competent at—I'd say, "My ability to see patterns and relationships." In this miraculous age of information overload, sorting through the noise of advertising, gimmickry, quick fixes, and fads taxes even what I believe to be my meager self-professed super-skill. And I've had training and experience—a lot of it. Thinking about restoring and optimizing the human condition is an all-out obsession for both me and those coaches and teachers in what my brilliant business partner and wife, Juliet, calls my "nerd cabal." So to say that even I sometimes find myself struggling to keep up with the fire hose of often conflicting and always varied health and wellness information out there makes me appreciate the potential Gordian knot that our friends and neighbors face when it comes to taking control over their long-term health.

On the face of it, the simple complexity of the human being is downright overwhelming. The human brain alone is the most sophisticated and complex structure in the known universe. Add that "machine" to the self-healing, tolerant, extraordinary, anti-fragile human body, and it's hard to know where to even begin. Oh, and we are complex psycho-emotional beings to boot! What I can tell you with 100 percent certainty is that a few pieces of information apply to you:

1. You have no idea of the depth of your physical capacities or resilience.
2. The resting state of the human is pain-free.
3. Your body is designed to function well over a lifetime that could easily last a hundred years.

I've spent decades in the trenches of the battle for human performance, and I believe unabashedly in these three statements. And what I've come also to believe is that you don't need a fancy coach, sleep tracker, protein shake, supplement, or degree in bio-hacking to benefit from what is your human birthright and inheritance. On the contrary, you simply need a different framework to see through all the noise and interference. Fortunately for you, you're holding it in your hands.

We have a saying around our house: "Show me you can be consistent before you are heroic." Consistency isn't sexy. Informed simplicity will never be "Insta-famous." One of the issues of being a modern human is that it's hard for us to appreciate how long a hundred years really is. Advanced medicine makes it much more likely that, barring catastrophe, most of us will make it to a significantly advanced age. The question this naturally begets is, "How capable do I want to be when I get there?" The flip side to this impending amortality is that who we are and what we do today dictates the experience on the back half of our lives.

Yes, our human physiology is remarkably tolerant, but no, it won't put up with our crap forever. It's confusing, I know. I have Olympic gold medalist friends who could eat a whole bag of little chocolate donuts, sneak a cigarette, pull an all-nighter, and still run rings around me on my best day. But I don't use this as an excuse to believe that my lifestyle doesn't matter. On the contrary, I take this extraordinary built-in human capacity as a sign that I don't have to get it right immediately, and that I can afford to not be perfect. It's never too late to make positive change. At what age again does your body stop healing? Oh, that's right. Never. The magic of this book is that Aaron has given us a template that we can begin to lay over our lives today, and one that will continue to work long, long into the future.

If you are obsessed with pattern recognition and understanding how things relate, then at some point you have to ask, "What is essential here?" If you talk to any of the greatest minds alive today about what would improve any output of human function and overall quality of life, most would agree that the lessons contained in these pages are the place to start. Most of my "deep nerd" friends would concur that the point of studying sports and human performance is so that we can apply lessons learned to the rest of our "mere mortal" selves and lives. In a not-insignificant twist of ironic fate, we are coming to realize that the first principles of being human aren't really that complicated or even that sexy: sleep, play, get out in sunlight, eat whole food, foster community, be active in nature, and, perhaps most important, move. Wash, rinse, repeat for the rest of your life.

You see, we tend to treat our health and wellness like a finite game. Such games have clear beginnings and ends, and the rules are clear to everyone. Infinite games, on the other hand, can't ever be "won." The rules are unclear (stress, disease, injury, life, children, work), and we aren't really sure when the game will end. The only way to win is to keep playing, and to play as well as you are able today. Tomorrow, you'll have a chance to play better. Now, if only you had some kind of primer, some sort of guidebook to make it easier to play your own infinite life game a little better, with more joy and less confusion. Aaron knows your body is extraordinary and he wants you to play beautifully. The game is on.

Kelly Starrett, DPT

THE
ALIGN METHOD

Introduction

"When your body is not aligned [形不正],
The inner power will not come.
When you are not tranquil within [中不靜],
Your mind will not be well ordered.
Align your body, assist the inner power [正形攝德],
Then it will gradually come on its own."

—*Ancient Chinese Guanzi Text (26 BCE)*

It's an ironic experience to walk into an event focusing on wellness and witness thousands of people hunching over their respective chairs, in an air-conditioned box, under beaming artificial lights, alternating between staring down at their cell phones and back up to the expert on stage pontificating on an illusory idea of optimal health. This scene would be confusing at best for our hunter-gatherer ancestors steeped in a more natural lifestyle that Westerners so often attempt to emulate. We are "standing on top of a whale while fishing for minnows," as Joseph Campbell said, and that whale is the way you move. Your vitality is determined by far more than overpriced supplements, complex dietary dogmas, or the latest fitness trends. The way you move impacts every aspect of your life and can be leveraged to make you feel stronger, more confident, and at home in your body.

The fundamentals of optimizing your life to move pain-free and feel your best are simple and teachable; this book contains the foundational principles for doing so. The collection of ideas within this book represent thousands of years of research from the world's preeminent thought leaders on all things movement and wellness to form the ultimate guide for physical inhabitance. What does that mean? Physical inhabitance is the way you sit, stand, walk, breathe, look, touch, listen, communicate, and generally occupy your body in any given moment during the day. It's a choice to either passively allow life to slip by or to actively engage in the ongoing process of growing into yourself. In the coming chapters, you will learn exactly how to leverage each moment of the day to become the strongest, sharpest, and most stress-proof version of yourself.

WHY I'M TELLING THIS STORY

I began my journey in a similar place as many young people: insecure and unsure how to feel confident in my own skin. Growing up with the body of a confused baby giraffe, a set of crooked teeth, and a bowl cut would be challenging for anyone, but things became especially interesting when my home life began deteriorating. Enter compensation in the form of fitness. I worked out relentlessly in a vain attempt to create a strong body to act as a fortress within chaos. When I was around age sixteen, it was no surprise to receive a call telling me my dad had finally been taken to prison on a slew of felony charges ranging from possession of crack cocaine to illegal weapons to prostitution. Before that call, the drugs had wreaked so much havoc that I would relentlessly rehearse in preparation for receiving a much bleaker message, so the news he had been locked up was oddly comforting.

In retrospect, this was the beginning of my interest in the way thoughts and emotions form our physical structures and, reciprocally, the power movement has to influence our mental, emotional, and physiological makeup. After several years of insulating myself with muscle by obsessing over bodybuilding in a variety of unhealthy ways, things finally began breaking down—I started to suffer from dislocating joints, chronic back pain, and an underlying, ineffable sensation of disconnect. My body appeared to be the peak expression of a fit male, yet internally I felt ashamed and out of place. It became clear something needed to change: I had been so focused on pushing for the most impressive-appearing exterior, I hadn't realized I was grinding myself down while simultaneously pushing others away. I needed to change the way I treated my body and re-form my definition of strength. It was time to stop pushing and start balancing. This eventually became the foundation for my work with clients, assisting them to find ease in their own bodies and gain relationship with themselves by accessing the power of their own movement.

The Align Method represents the tools and practices I've encountered over the past sixteen years of professionally seeking physical, mental, and emotional balance for myself and the amazing clients I've had the opportunity to work with. It isn't just reaffirming the traditional definitions of exercise, but rather is about how to merge movement awareness into daily life so each moment becomes an opportunity for greater alignment and vitality. It isn't a static method as much as it is an approach to life. Bruce Lee said "Set patterns, incapable of adaptability, of pliability, only offer a better cage. Truth is outside of all patterns." This is a principles-based field manual on occupying your body to burn fat, build muscle, increase energy levels, and move better as you grow older.

Where did the belief emerge that our bodies are constructed to inevitably break down with age? This is simply not true. Yes, these bodies are loaners, and we'll trade them in sooner or later, but the manner in which you age is a choice based on how you live today. The modern environment no longer naturally forms us into strong, flexible, aligned bodies—we need to pay special attention to lifestyle and movement function to be smarter than the misaligned modern world we occupy.

I'm warning you ahead of time: There will be aspects of the book that won't seem exactly "normal" or "comfortable." That's the whole point. The modern definition of "normal" is, for the most part, a state of imbalance. Long-term success is the product of making more balanced decisions on a momentary basis. Your movement and lifestyle could be compared to a golfer driving a ball: the subtlest of changes upon the moment of contact may not be immediately noticeable over the first few yards, but with time and distance traveled, those initial millimeters are the difference between the ball happily landing on the green or shanking into the rough. The standard club angle of modern culture is slightly askew, and this is an opportunity to readjust using the lessons to come in following chapters. The evolution of our species is dependent on those of us who are willing to be different, so be proud of your pursuit to think and move beyond the pale of normalcy.

Let's get started.

PART I

WELCOME TO YOUR BODY

CHAPTER 1

Stand Up for Yourself—Posture and Personality

"The way you walk through a room is the way you walk through life."
—Ida Rolf, founder of Rolfing Structural Integration

Your movement is literally an expression of the way in which you think and feel. Have you ever noticed a random guy approach a beautiful girl (or vice versa) in a coffee shop and curiously observed the dynamic? You can tell from across the room if he feels confident in his approach and simultaneously see if she believes he's a viable mate worthy of sharing her coveted digits with based purely on the dynamics of their movement. Is this because you've been endowed with telepathic superpowers, or could it be that you're reading their body language? A fascinating study conducted by researchers at Ohio State University showed how posture during communication not only informs the way others perceive you, but may even shape your own self-belief.[1] They asked study participants to list three positive and three negative traits they possess that would impact their professional performance at a future job. Half of the participants were asked to write these traits while they were in a hunched-over position, while the other half were asked to assume an upright posture during the process.

The results were striking. Their posture not only impacted whether or not they identified with the positive things they were asked to write about themselves, but also affected a participant's belief in the statements, positive or negative. That's right: A person's belief of their own words is associated with their postural position while thinking them. When you're in a hunched-over position, you may begin to distrust yourself, in the same way others would distrust the level of confidence in your statements.

Along with affecting the way you think about yourself, your postural patterns even impact the filter in which you access memories. A study conducted at San Francisco State University by professor of health education Erik Peper showed that more than 85 percent of the time, students found it easier to access uplifting memories in an upright (aligned) position and, reciprocally, easier to access depressive memories in a slumped posture.[2] Peper suggested, "You can take charge of yourself. Put yourself in an empowering, upright position. Remember that our thoughts and emotions are represented in our bodies. And vice versa: Our bodies can change our thoughts."

Throughout the book, I use "mind" and "body" as two separate words regularly: this is a limitation in language, not the reality of the human experience. In my career, I've yet to meet a person whose physical patterns did not relate to their history and personality or whose overall muscular tone did not match their temperament. If you're feeling tense or anxious, your muscles are tense and anxious. If you feel calm and relaxed, you can imagine the effect on your soft tissues. Here's a nice insight on trauma expressing itself in the body from one of the seminal books on this mind-body relationship, *The Body Keeps the Score*, by Bessel van der Kolk, MD:

Trauma victims cannot recover until they become familiar with and befriend the sensations in their bodies. Being frightened means you live in a body that is always on guard. Angry people live in angry bodies. The bodies of childhood victims are tense and offensive until they find a way to relax and feel safe. In order to change, people need to become aware of their sensations and the way that their bodies interact with the world around them. Physical self-awareness is the first step in releasing the tyranny of the past.[3]

Let's repeat that: "Physical self-awareness is the first step in releasing the tyranny of the past." Upon gaining a relationship with your physical experience, you are simultaneously taking steps to gain control of your mental and emotional self.

Your body has an immediate physical reaction to thoughts and experiences. This is a good thing: The problem arises when a traumatic experience causes the body to contract and the afflicted individual lacks the space, resources, or know-how to naturally reset their nervous system back to a baseline of homeostasis.

In the book *Waking the Tiger,* master somatic therapist Peter Levine discusses the natural responses various animals display after being immobilized by stress: They literally shake it off in a self-soothing process before getting back to their daily grind. Imagine a zebra just barely making it out of the clutches of a hungry lion: The stress of the situation needs to go somewhere after the escape. The tremors following the close call for the zebra are part of the process of discharging stress, a reboot for the nervous system bringing the frightened animal back to a healthy baseline. If the process is interrupted, Levine goes on to write, the stress is not released from the body, health problems will ensue, and the symptoms will not go away until the responses are discharged and the process of releasing the stress is completed.[4]

Humans, on the other hand, experience stressful "micro-traumas" each day in the form of rejection, noise pollution, minor accidents, the mechanical stress of moving with imbalanced postures, or anything that induces a sense of anxiety or fear in the organism. The short-term solution for many people is to keep pushing on instead of allowing a moment to fully shake off the newfound stress formed in the body, leaving their physiology assuming a lion is still hanging off their backs as they forge forward into the tasks of the day.

Most folks can make it through their lives with a few small lions (imbalanced postural patterns, financial, relationship, or environmental stressors, etc.) continually hanging on and slowly draining energy, but thankfully we have Starbucks (sarcasm) to keep us moving across the savanna (no wonder Americans spent $74.2 billion in 2015 on coffee alone).[5] If we don't pay attention to shaking these hungry carnivores off, they'll add up, and before we know it our precious bodies begin succumbing to postural collapse, sleep disruption, joint pain, unhealthy food cravings, dis–ease, and a mind partial to negative self-talk.

There's a solution to this: Shake these daily metaphoric lion attacks from your back as they happen instead of allowing them to add up and compromise your ability to maintain control of your own body. The principles outlined in the coming chapters will offer you the necessary tools to unravel the day's stressors via simple adjustments to your environment and subtle shifts in your physical inhabitance to shake any clinging lions (stressors) and prevent future attacks.

ALIGN YOURSELF

After something stressful takes place in your day (lion attack of any shape or size), take a beat to reset before entering into your next appointment, conversation, or event of the day. Call a time-out and observe yourself by slowly using this modification of a box-style breathing pattern: Breathe in for four seconds, hold for four seconds, breathe out for six seconds, hold for four seconds. Repeat this pattern six times. I've found the extra time breathing out assists in down-regulating the nervous system into a calmer state than the traditional four-by-four-by-four-by-four-style box breathing. Compound the stress-reducing variables by taking a walk outside as you follow the breath practice. For bonus destressing points, feel free to jump, wiggle, vibrate, twist, and turn your body while you're on your walk.

MOVING YOUR PHYSIOLOGY

"It's easier to act your way into a new way of thinking than to think your way into a new way of acting."
—Millard Fuller, founder of Habitat for Humanity

Now, where the conversation gets intriguing is when we realize our postural patterns appear to have deep physiological ramifications. It's as though our endocrine system is deciphering our postural positions like a person reading braille and actually changing our mood based on the signaling of our movement.

It appears your hormones may act like messengers between your postural patterns and the state you experience. A trio of social psychology professors—Amy Cuddy from Harvard, Andy Nap from Yale, and Dana Carney from the University of California, Berkeley—explored this idea in 2010 when they popularized the idea of "high-power poses," which were shown to boost levels of testosterone by around 20 percent and reduce cortisol (a stress hormone) levels by 25 percent after spending just two minutes in them. Inversely, the researchers found that "low-power poses" (e.g., hunching over to scroll on your phone) increased cortisol levels and decreased testosterone.[6] This study was a testament to the speed at which the body is continually processing postural information into chemical stimuli: Your cells are always listening.

In Cuddy's TED Talk (at the date of writing, the second most viewed one of all time), she describes the power of "faking it until you make it," suggesting that you can literally change the way you feel and behave based upon the way you organize your physical body.[7] This particular study has gone through an immense amount of scrutiny, in large part due to its popularity. A paper came out in 2017 refuting Cuddy's findings,[8] and then another in 2018 reaffirmed the concept referred to as "postural feedback."[9] At this point, it's fairly indisputable that the way you move (or don't) affects the way you feel, and the way you feel is inseparably tied to the expression of your internal chemistry. Envision a weight lifter hyping themselves up before stepping onto a platform or a UFC fighter strutting into an octagon as a display of dominance. Research on these miraculous moments can be challenging because life doesn't happen in a controlled, double-blind, static, sterile laboratory setting, and thus these debates will likely continue.

An issue with *faking* a powerful pose does arise when the focus is solely on the upper body — the trick is to find alignment (power) from feet to head. When people pull their shoulders back to pretend a power pose, they typically end up jamming their low back into an unstable hyperlordotic (or overly arched) position that is unfortunately not very powerful at all. It can create the appearance of confident readiness but will not be stable or sustainable without a strong foundation of regular full-body integration—as the body neutralizes back to its habituated posture, the confidence boost you wanted recedes, too. Throughout this book, you will learn the fundamental movement and lifestyle practices to create long-term structural change in your body so there's nothing to fake, and you can feel strong and confident from the ground up.

ALIGN YOURSELF

If you're anything like me, you'll find it a bit funny to stand like Wonder Woman for a couple of minutes contemplating how awesome you are. Instead, try hanging from a pull-up bar, jungle gym, or even a strong tree branch to lengthen your body into the same position. This will give you the gratification of restoring optimal shoulder function (more on this in Chapter 7), while also creating an emotional pick-me-up. Remember, hanging can be playful; if you're physically able, make a point to climb a tree or jungle gym every now and again. Allow yourself to enjoy a little childlike movement and remember to smile, because that too profoundly improves your physiological state!

DO YOU SPEAK MOVEMENT?

"Our bodies are apt to be our autobiographies."

—Frank Gillette Burgess

You've almost certainly heard the term "body language," but have you ever really thought its meaning through? Turns out, we communicate with each other nonverbally all the time. UCLA professor Albert Mehrabian coined the famous 7/38/55 ratio of our communication back in the seventies, showing that most of what we *say* to each other is actually conveyed via our body language and the tonality of our voice rather than the words themselves.[10] Mehrabian found about 55 percent of our communication is body language, 38 percent is voice tonality, and only 7 percent is conveyed through the literal words spoken.[11]

This is obviously difficult to quantify exactly, and Mehrabian himself cautioned that his experiments were limited to feelings and attitudes, particularly when there were incongruences: If the body language and words disagree, one will tend to trust the body. Thus, closely observing what your body is *saying* is wise if you care about clearly expressing yourself.

Learning to speak more effectively with your movement will not only make you a better orator, it may very well save your life (or at least your wallet) someday. In a study from 1981, researchers Betty Grayson and Morris I. Stein asked criminals convicted of violent offenses to watch a video of pedestrians walking down a busy city sidewalk and point out who would be a likely target. It only took seconds to point the potential victims out, and the results were consistent among all the convicts. What were the patterns these clueless pedestrians were exhibiting, you ask?

It wasn't their race, gender, age, or even size—it was the way in which they moved! Researchers determined it was nonverbal cues such as their pace of walking, length of stride, posture, body language, and awareness of the environment. One of the primary precipitators of attracting unwanted attention from a predator is a walking style lacking what researchers called "wholeness"— what we refer to in this book as integration.[12] If your body appears disorganized in the way you move, it's perceived as weakness and makes you more likely to be exploited. That's why realigning your movement is so important: Balancing your body parts allows you to exude strength and confidence, attracting the right people into your life and dispelling the wrong ones, even when you don't realize it's happening.

Move the way you want to feel. This is a three-step process that will take some thinking outside of the traditional box for some.

Step one: Think about how you would like to feel. It could be strong, confident, humble, graceful, powerful, flexible, aggressive, humorous, light, or anything of the sort.

Step two: Visualize the way your body moves when you feel this way, and be specific. Notice how your arms and legs swing when you walk, how you sit, stand, breathe, communicate, and even the tone and pace of your voice.

Step three: Take a walk and explore moving in the way you just visualized. How does it feel? Start actively thinking about moving more this way as often as is reasonable, choose sports or activities that promote this style of movement, and begin to notice how your postural patterns affect the way you think and feel.

FACIAL FLEXIBILITY

If your overall posture affects how you feel, what do all of those face muscles do? Have you ever thought about why you have such a complex facial structure continually contorting into all those strange positions? It has something to do with that 55 percent of our communication coming from body language: As most would agree, a single facial expression really can tell a thousand words. Paul Ekman, emeritus professor of psychology at the University of California, San Francisco, has spent more than forty years exploring this topic all across the globe. In a past podcast episode, he and I discussed how he found humans to utilize more than 10,000 facial expressions in conversation, all with subtle and specific meanings.[13] The forty-three muscles of the face have an exponential capacity to convey distinct messages—more honestly than the actual words coming out of your mouth.

Take, for example, the vast difference in meaning between a diabolical, expressionless smile involving only the muscles around the mouth (zygomatic major muscles) compared to a person gleaming with their eye muscles as well (orbicularis oculi). This more honest-appearing smile is referred to as the Duchenne smile, named after the French anatomist Guillaume Duchenne, and is sometimes referred to as "smizing," as in smiling with your eyes. It sends the signal you are safe and honest; a smile without the eyes tells people you may be faking it and up to something suspicious.

So what does this mean for plastic surgery? you may be thinking. In one study using functional magnetic resonance imaging (fMRI) scans, researchers discovered less activation in areas of the brain used to interpret and modulate emotional states in people who had had Botox injections. This means your facial expressions are like emotional conductors, and your ability to play your own internal orchestra of sensation is associated to your facial (and postural) mobility.[14] This phenomenon is referred to as the "facial feedback hypothesis" and suggests the control of facial expression produces parallel effects on subjective feelings. This suggests that in order to empathize with another human being, it's helpful to literally form yourself to the shape of their present state to truly feel for them.

That's right, even empathy could be likened to a form of fitness—greater movement competence through a wider range of postural and facial expressions allows a person to connect more deeply to a broader population, because each person moves a little bit differently. If you can match your movement expression to another's like a key in a lock, they will feel seen and felt by you. This gives new meaning to Louis Armstrong's iconic song lyric "When you're smiling, the whole world smiles with you," although perhaps "when you're smizing, the whole world smizes with you" may lead to a more joyous outcome.

Are these facial expressions universally consistent, indicating the way you move your muscles to express emotion is not learned, but rather is integrated deep into human psychobiology? Charles Darwin was convinced our facial expressions were distinct to each culture, but Paul Ekman was not. He traveled to Papua New Guinea in the late sixties to visit the Fore people, a tribe without any exposure to outside influence. Just as Ekman anticipated, their expressions were interpreted the same way as they would be by any Westerner. This is yet another example of our postural expression underlying the superficial accoutrements of spoken language. Your movement is the mainframe of effective communication and largely defines your own inner self-talk.

EXPAND YOUR BODY LANGUAGE VOCABULARY

"Preach the gospel at all times. When necessary, use words."

—*St. Francis*

The same way reading or spending time with people who communicate using vernacular beyond what you're accustomed will expand your vocabulary, think about expanding your movement "vocabulary" by pursuing activities like dancing, yoga, Pilates, weight lifting, theater, martial arts, or any other form of physical expression. As you grow your movement literacy, you can learn the fundamental patterns, or grammar, of organizing these "words" so they give your body the full range of communication. You can think of the 5 Daily Movements section of this book (Part II) to be like staple words to integrate into your daily "speech," and the overarching principles consistent throughout the chapters to be the grammar holding all the words together.

POSTURAL ARCHETYPES

"A purely disembodied human emotion is a nonentity."

—*William James*

You can usually assess a person's mood by looking at their posture, and you can even alter your own state by simply changing the shape of the way you stand.

William James, often referred to as the father of American psychology, famously proposed that emotional experiences are perceptions of bodily processes. What the heck does that mean? He described it this way: "Common sense says, we lose our fortune, are sorry and weep; we meet a bear, are frightened and run; we are insulted by a rival, are angry and strike. The hypothesis here to be defended says that this order of sequence is incorrect, that the one mental state is not immediately induced by the other, that the bodily manifestations must first be interposed between, and that the more rational statement is that we feel sorry because we cry, angry because we strike, afraid because we tremble, and not that we cry, strike, or tremble because we are sorry, angry, or fearful, as the case may be. Without the bodily states following on the perception, the latter would be purely cognitive in form, pale, colourless, destitute of emotional warmth. We might then see the bear, and judge it best to run, receive the insult and deem it right to strike, but we could not actually feel afraid or angry."

James hypothesized this idea before seeing the present-day research that shows how simply holding a pencil in a person's teeth to induce a mechanical smile engenders a sensation of happiness[15] and furrowing someone's brow into the shape of a frown with a golf tee gives rise to sadness.[16] That's not to mention the effect temporary facial paralysis (e.g., Botox), as discussed previously, may have on a person's ability to fully interpret and feel emotions. (Side note: This chapter is clearly biased toward physical movement being a primary catalyst for one's internal experience. Evidence and logic suggests it's a two-way relationship—in Chapter 18, on mindfulness, we will dive deeper into how one's internal state shapes their physical structure.)

Let's now take a look at the five most common postural archetypes. We will detail them from an anatomical perspective and describe the personality type most commonly associated with each postural pattern. The majority of people will identify with a combination of the archetypes, with one or two standing out most prominently. Every person has the opportunity to find greater alignment in themselves by following the steps outlined in the coming chapters.

Archetype 1: Mopey

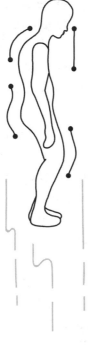

The Mopey person typically moves with low energy and appears structurally as though their body is being pulled to the ground. This position is typically associated with feeling sad, disconnected, tired, or dare I say depressed. Depression has proliferated to become the number one leading cause of disability worldwide. This frightening trend is happening in tandem with our collapsed postural tendencies, as we become more and more pulled-down to stare at devices and spend hours sitting in the same chronically collapsed positions.

Is there a postural connection to this mental health epidemic? I'm personally not attached to either a bottom-up (body affects the mind) or top-down (mind affects the body) perspective on the topic, as it seems apparent each side reciprocally interacts with the other. Movement and postural patterns are keys to mental and emotional well-being (and vice versa)—it's wise to pay attention to all the factors at play for optimal development.

Structurally speaking, this state can be broken down anatomically to medial rotation of the shoulders, hyperkyphosis of the thoracic spine (where the spine curves forward, leading to a rounding of the upper back), forward head posture manifesting as a "righting reflex" to counter the hunched-over spine, pelvis tucking under like a dog who knows he did something wrong, knees buckling inward (valgus), feet collapsing inward (pronation), and the facial muscles lowering the corners of the mouth while raising the inner portion of the eyebrows. As a result, the Mopey person looks and feels a bit flat, as though the world is literally pulling them down.

MOVEMENT TIP: *Doorway Stretch*

Start by standing in a tall, proud, and upright position beside a doorway. Guide your breath into the side of your lower ribs and belly to feel the diaphragm engaging to move your breath and calm your nervous system. Imagine you're attempting to grow your arms down to the ground so your shoulders lengthen away from your ears, and then begin raising one arm up toward the edge of the doorway, while maintaining the length you just created in your neck and shoulders. Grab the edge of the doorway with your raised hand and slowly rotate your body and head away from the outstretched hand, creating a stretch through the shoulder and neck. (Visit TheAlignBook.com for a detailed video guide to this and other movements.)

If you're feeling down, start looking for movements that will focus on opening, straightening, and awakening your body. Consider some sweaty dance classes with upbeat music, aerobic exercise, hot yoga to loosen up tight muscles, or resetting the system with a plunge in an icy lake (or cold shower), summiting a mountain (or a local hill), or restructuring and strengthening your body with some weight lifting (kettlebell swings, squats, and dead lifts, etc.) Think about taking up more space with your body instead of shrinking inward, as this, too, has been shown to induce a greater sense of confidence.

Archetype 2: Anxious

This person can be spotted with their shoulders up, as if attempting to have an affair with their ears. Their eyes are peeled wide open anticipating impact, their mouth may be dry, and the breath is short and predominantly in the upper chest as a response to their nervous system bracing to fight, flight, or freeze to protect against a potential predator (modern "predators" include bills, deadlines at work, stressful relationships, etc.). Issues they might deal with include high anxiety driving their blood pressure up, chronically elevated cortisol, and digestive issues.

The Anxious archetype tends to be more high-strung, preferring to keep moving at all times, and will

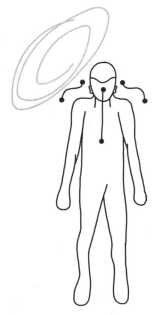

have tightly wound muscles to match. Their neck and shoulders are chronically carrying excess tension and their breath is short, mostly coming from the chest and neck muscles. The pace of walking and talking is fast and tends to make other people feel a bit on edge because of it.

MOVEMENT TIP: *Gut Massage*

Your guts are considered to be your "second brain": If they're tense, that sensation will ripple through your whole nervous system, leaving you feeling the same. You can use a resistance band (I recommend the Align Band because it includes a door anchor to adjust the height of the hanging band) to lightly massage your abdomen while intentionally breathing into the areas of tension by placing the door anchor at chest height and wrapping it around your abdomen. Step forward to create tension in the band and roll your spine downward so the band creates a subtle "flossing" effect on your guts. Try breathing out a few seconds longer than you breathe in, and explore making an auditory *uhhh* sound as you exhale to help relax the tense tissues. (You can jump ahead to Chapter 16 for more on the therapeutic effects of sound.)

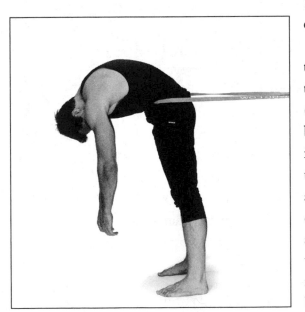

Keys for unwinding the tension may include massage therapy, organic essential oils (especially lavender, which has been shown to have a calming effect), time in nature, and taking fun movement classes of any kind. Steer clear of overly caffeinated beverages and high amounts of sugar. Instead drink warm, calming teas and pop a magnesium supplement to relax before bed.

Archetype 3: Swole

This pattern is near and dear to my heart because it's exactly where I came from, as you read in the introduction. These people (usually male) feel the need to present themselves as being strong and dominant so other people know they're in control. Think of a gorilla pounding its chest to let the other beta males know he's the top sexual prospect. The interesting part about going out of your way to signal to other people how strong you are is that it usually stems from a place of insecurity. If you truly feel strong, powerful, and in control of your life, there's not much reason to search for validation by beating your chest about it.

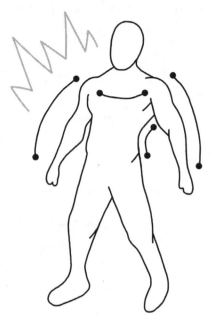

Anatomically, this pattern appears to be pretty balanced from chest to head, with the shoulders rolled back, neck long for the head to raise higher, and palms slightly front facing (supinated) to signal to the world to bring it on. The imbalances in this position are stuffed down into the lower back (where people can't see the instability the person is experiencing—oh, the metaphors). This causes the ribs to flare open, reducing abdominal integrity, and encourages chest breathing that puts the person in a continual fight-or-flight state. The legs of the Swole person will tend to point a bit outward (externally rotated) and the gait pattern is a combination of a waddle and strut with the chest puffed out—stiff as if a stick has been carefully shoved up their butt (with love, of course).

MOVEMENT TIP: *Dynamic Spinal Twists and Hand Slaps*

This is a fabulous way to warm up your body and circulate lymphatic fluid that can build up throughout the day. Here's what you do: Stand up tall and rotate your spine left and right, allowing your hands to swing and slap the opposite shoulders. Work your hands down your body giving each side a healthy splash of slap therapy. This is a powerful tool to loosen yourself up before any athletic event or to just start the day.

I would also recommend spending more time floating and swimming to help loosen up the body and mind. Complement more water time with some partner dance to soften enough to connect with another person in rhythm, and the Swole person will begin feeling even more comfortable in their own skin.

Archetype 4: Bendy

The Bendy person loves all things about mobility but tends to avoid strength development because it's not as much fun. This type is typically very kind but can sometimes be a bit of a pushover. They will generally go with the flow of things and try not to ruffle too many feathers. Sometimes the Bendy person runs behind on time because they tend to become lost in the moment with what's in front of them. This person may be a bit spacey but is very creative; they could use a more stable and grounded friend to help organize and actualize their ideas.

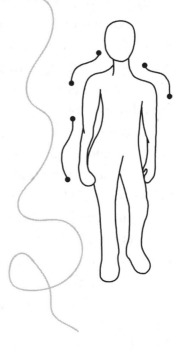

Anatomically, the Bendy archetype is, well, bendy. This sounds good, and it can be; the issue comes when a person lacks stability. They tend to lean toward activities that lend themselves to even greater flexibility, such as yoga, and they may also be seen at a local ecstatic dance. Their connective tissue feels very loose to the touch, with a few areas chronically tight to help balance out the excessive mobility elsewhere. They can greatly benefit from weight lifting, manual labor, greater core stability, and a focus on active mobility instead of passive (discussed in Chapter 3).

MOVEMENT TIP: *Slowly and Safely Add Weight Lifting to Your Movement Practice*

Begin introducing dead lifts and/or back squats to your workout one to two times per week. (Follow the principles outlined in Chapter 6 and/or get a knowledgeable coach to guide you through the lifts; it's worth it.) Try five sets of five reps to start: The first sets can be light just to practice the motion, and you can gradually move up to about 90 percent of maximum (or to the weight under which you can still maintain perfect form) by the fifth set. Take a three-to-five-minute break between sets in which you work on something else or just take a walk.

If weight lifting isn't your thing, I recommend manual labor such as carpentry, landscaping, or anything that gets your hands dirty while moving weight. The gratification of stepping back and looking at something you built with your own hands will be helpful.

Archetype 5: Aligned

Some say depression is focusing too much on the past and anxiety is focusing too much on the future. There is a middle ground between these two points, and it's where the Aligned person spends most of their time. You won't see them jutting their heads forward looking into what's to come or drooping back wishing the good ol' days were here again. Instead, they're thriving in the present moment with exactly what life has dealt them, be it hard or easy. They embody Shakespeare's idea of there being no such thing as good or bad, and our thoughts making it so, and thus feel a sense of balance no matter what the circumstance.

The Aligned person appears tall and strong no matter their height; you could draw a plumb line down from their ears to their shoulders, hips, knees, and ankles. They're light on their feet and seem to gain energy as they move instead of wearing down and becoming more tired with every step in a slow journey of attrition. The tonicity of the Aligned person's muscles is supple at rest, and they can snap into activation at a moment's notice. They naturally tire as it gets dark

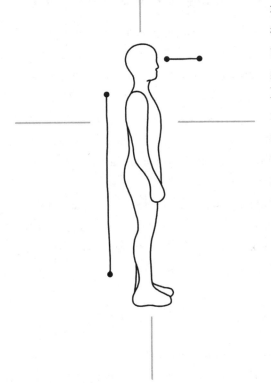

and wake up full of energy as the sun rises. They do well in social situations, and people tend be magnetized toward them because they exude a healthy glow. German-American poet Charles Bukowski once said, "The free soul is rare but you know it when you see it—basically you feel good, very good when you are near or with them." By free soul, I think he was referring to the Aligned person.

Once the mind and body have transitioned into an aligned state and the environment has been formed to match it, the person will naturally become healthier simply by living their lives. This is what Ida Rolf, the founder of Rolfing Structural Integration, meant when she wrote, "This is the gospel of Rolfing: when the body gets working appropriately, the force of gravity can flow through. Then, spontaneously the body heals itself."

The Aligned person will remain humble and lead others into better alignment via their own positive example. They don't feel the need to shame or criticize others for living different lifestyles. They monitor and cultivate their thoughts because they realize perception is of greater value than circumstances, and thus this person typically feels balanced and equanimous.

MOVEMENT TIP: *Activate Your Senses*

The Aligned person likely already naturally does the 5 Daily Movements (floor sitting, nasal breathing, hip hinging, hanging, and walking) with regularity, so I recommend focusing on Part IV: Moving Your Senses to bringing more healthy movement into your life via the power of sight, sound, touch, and mindfulness.

ALIGN YOURSELF

Grab a piece of paper (or feel free to write in the book; I won't be offended) and label the sensation and characteristics of your major joints and appendages. Write out a couple adjectives for each, starting with your feet, then ankles, knees, hips, spine, shoulders, head, neck, elbows, and hands. This list will contain around twenty words ranging from strong, stable, rough, quiet, clear, rigid, dependable to loose, flexible, open, expansive, loud, unstable, bright, or whatever comes to mind. Now that you have your list, notice whether it's an accurate description of your personality and sense of the way you feel. See if you align with one postural archetype more than others, and after following along with the 5 Daily Movements for one month, come back and make the list again to see how it changes!

Alignment Assignment

Identify which postural archetype you relate to most, and begin incorporating the Movement Tip associated with the archetype into your life this week. If the movement feels good, keep doing it!

Also, start noticing the way people move and the how it relates to their personalities. For example, a great way to make your airport time more interesting is to actively observe people's postural patterns and play with creating a story of what they do, hobbies they enjoy, and see if you can relate a postural archetype to them as well. (The story you create may be way off. Just have fun with it.)

CHAPTER 2

Rigidity Tends to Break—Play May Save Your Brain and Body

"We don't stop playing because we get old, we get old because we stop playing."

—George Bernard Shaw

"Notice that the stiffest tree is most easily cracked, while the bamboo or willow survives by bending with the wind." So said martial arts master Bruce Lee. And yet while a child's fondness for unstructured play makes them like the supple bamboo or willow, most of us adults started becoming brittle like the stiff tree the moment we stopped playing and got serious. As a result, we not only stagnate but also leave ourselves open to becoming broken by our very rigidity.

In neuroscience, one of the hottest topics in the past few years has been neuroplasticity—i.e., the ability of the brain to be malleable, grow, and change. Your body is an extension of your brain, and a supple body represents a supple mind. Adaptability is the human's most valuable quality, necessary for the evolution of the species, and group play is the highest expression of instantaneous physical, cognitive, and emotional adaptability. Interactive play literally tones your autonomic nervous system, enhancing the capacity of your social engagement system to regulate reactions to future stressors. What the heck does that mean? It helps you become more resilient to stress and seamless in the way your nervous system switches gears between states. If a person "doesn't play well with others," it's an indication their nervous system is *stuck* in a defensive or shut-down state, and gradual exposure to playful social engagement can be just the remedy for bringing them back to balance. Looking through this lens, you could say play is the top of the movement food chain.

There may be some muscle-bound folks who find this statement challenging to hear. But think about the level of physical and cognitive engagement involved in a child running, jumping, climbing, twisting, turning, hinging, rolling, falling, rising, and bounding, all the while delving deep into his or her imagination (I personally was a big fan of becoming a Power Ranger, the blue one specifically). What muscle is this child using to joyfully play tag with friends or jump into a pile of leaves while howling with laughter? Answer: All of them! If this experience were a "movement supplement," it would be the mack daddy of all full-spectrum, organic, whole superfoods money can buy, and it would include all your macros and micros in one shot. (See the complexities of play that bely its apparent simplicity in the infographic on page 28.)

Children don't move well merely because they're kids, but because they've yet to be corrupted by long days of chair sitting followed by isolating their muscles with misaligned workouts. Practice doesn't make perfect, it simply imprints what you repeat—whether beneficial or not.

Excessive isolation of the parts will begin to disassemble the whole. I learned this all too well after injuring myself from years of bodybuilding incorrectly. Since then, my life has been a rewarding (and challenging) journey of putting the parts back together mentally, emotionally, and physically. My personal path back toward balance has drawn from relearning how to play in the form of sport, dance, martial arts, hiking, climbing, yoga of various varieties, weight lifting, and general movement exploration. During this exploration, it's become crystal clear to me that you can access the mind and emotions from the physical body via movement.

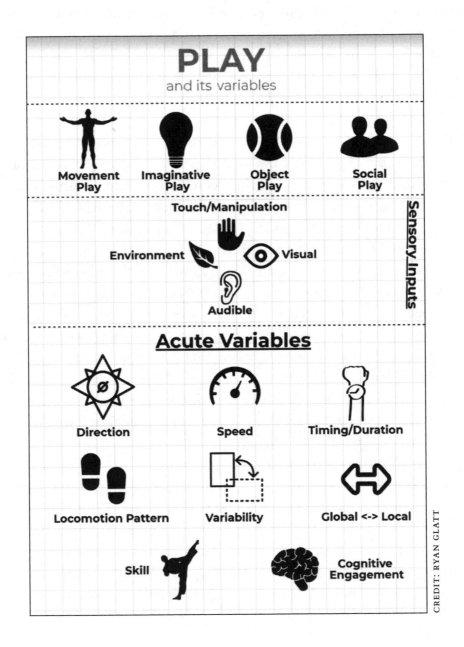

DO WHAT COMES NATURALLY

If, like me, you binge watch those brilliant BBC documentaries like *Planet Earth*, *The Life of Birds*, or *Blue Planet* the moment they hit Netflix, you'll know that playfulness isn't unique to human beings—it's universal across the animal kingdom. Chimps monkey around in games of hide-and-seek, crows slide down icy slopes, and hippos do backflips. Even insects like ants engage in play fighting. Some creatures, such as dolphins, seem to do little else but play.

So what's going on here? Why do animals play? Writing in a special edition of the journal *Current Biology*, Richard W. Byrne suggests, "Fun is functional: play is evolution's way of making sure animals acquire and perfect valuable skills in circumstances of relative safety." Connecting the dots back to our species, Byrne goes on to write, "For humans, the development of creativity may be another important functional explanation for why play is fun: building an enhanced mental repertoire, by exploring and linking concepts that might never occur together in real-life situations."[1]

This means we should do things outside the norm once in a while. In this age of hacks, we can get so caught up in trying to squeeze every ounce of productivity out of each day that we shun anything that doesn't help us to "optimize" (or insert your buzzword of choice). Yet when we choose to embrace novelty and—like those silly chimps hiding their faces behind big leaves—be silly for its own sake, we have the chance to develop new skills, enhance our interaction with others, and come up with new ways to express ourselves.

ALIGN YOURSELF

Add a few animal movements, such as bear crawls or lizard crawls, to your workout for a five-minute warm-up, or make up your own fun way to move on the ground as a way to open your hips, and engage your hands and shoulders while taking yourself less seriously. Visit www.TheAlign Book.com to see a video tutorial on how to perform the techniques!

PLAYING THE BRAIN GAME

Over a hundred years ago, Maria Montessori, the founder of the Montessori education movement, wrote, "One of the greatest mistakes of our day is to think of movement by itself. As something apart from the higher functions. Mental development must be connected with movement and be dependent on it. Watching a child makes it obvious that the development of his mind comes through his movements. Mind and movement are part of the same entity." In Montessori schools, children learn grammar and vocabulary by acting out sentences and learn the alphabet by tracing letters for an embodied learning experience. Your brain does not exist in a vacuum; it's not a part of your body, it *is* your body. By incorporating playful movement into activities focusing on cognitive development, you're able to create more meaningful associations with the ideas being presented. I like to think of the brain-body like a sponge absorbing liquid—if it's dry and stiff, it will repel new fluid. If it's soft and malleable, it's able to receive.

A study published in *Frontiers in Psychology* demonstrated that unstructured play such as free-drawing or imaginative play (e.g., role playing or roughhousing) free of rules and guidelines improves executive functions like focus, organization, task initiation, and keeping track of what you're doing. Unsupervised playtime also improved participants' ability to keep their emotions on an even keel.[2] Furthermore, the work of Estonian neuroscientist Jaak Panksepp demonstrated that as little as half an hour of movement-based play modified at least a third of the 1,200 brain genes assessed by Northwestern University's Falk Center for Molecular Therapeutics.[3]

In his book *Play*, Stuart Brown reveals that play doesn't just stimulate us at a genetic level or merely excite existing neurons in the brain, it actually creates new cells—a process called neurogenesis. It links up certain areas of the brain like rangers joining trails in a national park. "Play also promotes the creation of new connections that didn't exist before between neurons and between disparate brain centers," he writes. "It is activated from and organizes what I call 'divinely superfluous neurons.' These are neural connections that don't seem to have an immediate function but when fired up by play are, in fact, essential to continued brain organization."[4] It appears the creativity boost and ideation inspired by play actually ignites a mysterious realm of the mind only available to those willing to drop their guard enough to experience the occasional bout of unadulterated wonderment. The modern computer, for example, began as a device for gaming, and the gunpowder used by militaries to shape history originated from fireworks in China. You could say the world as we know it has been constructed upon the shoulders of playful exploration.

Play isn't just Miracle-Gro for the birth of novel ideas—it's an invaluable asset in maintaining a healthy mind throughout your entire life. A team of Polish, British, and German researchers whose work focuses on the physical and cognitive effects of aging showed when older adults get together to play, their minds and bodies benefit. "Engagement in playful pastime activities such as a game of Italian bocce, English lawn bowls, Spanish skittles or Polish sztekiel, in a socially valuable setting, can make a real difference to the emotional and cognitive engagement of older adults," the study authors wrote.[5]

As Albert Einstein urged, "Do not grow old. No matter how long you live. Never cease to stand like curious children before the great mystery into which we were born."

ALIGN YOURSELF

Your kids still have healthy hips in large part because they spend so much time moving from the ground and in foundational positions such as a lunge or squat while hinging from the hips. Take a page out of their book and get down there! If you have kids, grandkids, younger siblings, or little cousins, get down on the floor with them, tip out a giant box of Legos, and go to town. Think of this time playing on the ground like a brain-body massage!

STOP STRESS IN ITS TRACKS

How many articles have you seen about stress this week? Quite a few, I'll bet. Like you, I'm getting pretty tired of getting yet another top ten tips to relax, but we keep seeing them for a reason—the frenetic pace of our society is conducive to being anxious and wound up, not to mention the effect of our technology addiction (see the *South Park* clip of Eric Cartman yelling at everyone that he has anxiety issues while being permanently glued to his phone). Indeed, recent research cited by *Psychology Today* found that 90 percent of Generation Z-ers surveyed reported symptoms of chronic stress.[6]

The easiest solution—other than simplifying our calendars, cutting down on commitments, and taking more frequent tech breaks—might also be the most elemental: play. A review of research that has investigated the link between emotional state and play concluded, "Playful individuals reported lower levels of perceived stress than their less playful counterparts, and more frequently utilized adaptive, stressor-focused coping strategies and were less likely to employ negative, avoidant, and escape-oriented strategies."[7]

The University of Illinois at Urbana-Champaign researchers added that play might be particularly useful to those stressed out Generation Z-ers I mentioned a moment ago: "The results suggested that playfulness serves a strong adaptive function with university students, providing them with specific cognitive resources from which they can manifest effective coping behaviors in the face of stressful situations."[8]

ALIGN YOURSELF

If you're a college student, take advantage of those Ping-Pong and pool tables in the dorm, take every opportunity to toss a Frisbee or throw a football with your friends on the campus lawn, and sign up for a new activity you've never tried before in intramurals. Try a martial arts class, like jiujitsu or aikido. Chances are it won't just help your social life, but also boost your GPA and keep your stress levels at bay.

GAME YOUR NERVOUS SYSTEM

When I feel the need to geek out about the nervous system, one of the first things I check is if Dr. Stephen Porges has written any new articles. This psychiatry professor at the University of North Carolina devised what's known as polyvagal theory to explain the three levels of the autonomic nervous system. Porges believes that it's possible to enter a hybrid state that's somewhere between the social engagement system and the fight/flight/freeze response utilizing sensuality or—you guessed it!—play. "Play functions as a neural exercise that improves the efficiency of the neural circuit that can instantaneously down regulate fight/flight behaviors," Porges writes in a paper entitled "Play as a Neural Exercise: Insights into Polyvagal Theory."[9]

He goes on to state that while playing with toys or a computer may have certain benefits, it isn't as effective as engaging in a game with another human being, which allows us to tap into "a social engagement system that evolved to employ cues from face-to-face interactions to efficiently calm our physiological state and shift our fight/flight behaviors to trusting relationships." Porges goes on to say movement-based competitive play is the most effective, as it not only involves face-to-face interaction and playfulness, but also requires us to modulate our impulses and avoid losing control and lapsing into uncontrolled, violent rage.

Social engagement encourages our bodies to get back into a rest-digest parasympathetic recovery state. Getting together to play with movement kills the proverbial two birds with one stone (I vote we collectively change that phrase to "feed two birds with one hand," just saying), with both the social and play-based elements of movement-focused group activity improving brain health and elevating emotional and physical well-being.

ALIGN YOURSELF

A fun trick to "hack" your autonomic nervous system to make you feel more relaxed and social at the same time is to mobilize your facial muscles!

Try this technique when you're feeling stressed or before you are about to be tossed into a social situation you don't feel totally prepared for (yet). Place your fingers above your eyebrows and subtly lift the tissue upward with your fingers as you open and close all your facial muscles. Alternate from wide open to tightly closed for five seconds in 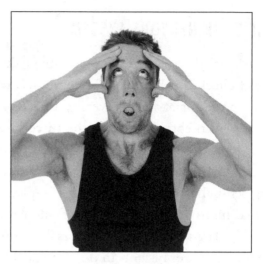 each position and repeat two to three times. For an added stress-easing effect, emphasize longer, fuller exhalations than inhalations, and to make it extra impactful (and let's face it, a little weird) you could exhale with a sigh.

LEARN, UNLEARN, RELEARN

"The illiterate of the 21st century will not be those who cannot read and write, but those who cannot learn, unlearn, and relearn."

—*Alvin Toffler*

Stew on this for a moment: We spend our most developmental years hunched over a desk under artificial lights, in tight, unventilated schools and buildings, in an overly synthetic, chemically sterilized environment, and repeat the same debilitating pattern in college and many typical workplaces.

I understand that's a very dismal picture to paint, but there is hope! We often hear kids need more PE, and I agree, but this isn't just an issue of volume—we also need to be teaching kids the art and science of physical inhabitance in daily life. The topic of *physical education* is far larger than the rules of basketball and soccer; it should teach students how to physically engage and care for their bodies to sustain themselves throughout their lives.

You learn with your whole body, not just your eyes and ears. If a student is habituating herself to a hunched-over, tired posture, she will not be primed to learn new information and/or think creatively to do something meaningful with the information. Just think for a moment about your own posture when you're eager to learn or receive a gift. Do you shrink up and hunch forward (me for most of my high school experience) or do you open your chest, pull your head and shoulders back, and open your postural patterns to take it all in? You could think of your posture like a valve you can open and close at your command to allow the "flow" of your outside world in or shut it out. If you're interested in what you're learning, open up and bring it in. Don't like what you see? Feel free to close down to shut it out (you'll do this subconsciously anyway).

In the coming chapters, I'm going to share with you some of the best movement medicine I've come across over the years, and a lot of it is inspired by the importance of play. Some of the techniques or exercises might make you feel silly, and that's OK—some of them are! But give yourself permission to have fun, to feel joy, to open your mind and body to new experiences. Movement isn't something that should be relegated to an hour a day on a machine or a few hours a week in a studio—it's the foundation of how you experience your life. So if you want to relieve stress, reduce pain, or increase confidence, the coming chapters will provide you some solutions!

Alignment Assignment

Take a lesson from children and begin observing the world through the lens of play. Simple acts such as jumping up to swing from a tree branch like your ancestors or opting to kick a can you notice on the street like a soccer player (ideally recycling it afterward) will add up to brain-body boosting momentum in the short and long term. There are more opportunities in your day to be playful than you think, and taking advantage of them will be restorative for your mind and body and perhaps even wake up your spirit!

CHAPTER 3

Tools and Techniques to Align Your Body

"All parts of the body which have a function, if used in moderation and exercised in labors in which each is accustomed, become thereby healthy, well developed and age more slowly, but if unused they become liable to disease, defective in growth and age quickly."

—*Hippocrates, regarded as the father of medicine*

GETTING TO KNOW YOUR BODY

We all grew up learning about muscles, tendons, ligaments, and bones, but few of us received much education on the stuff tying it all together: the fibrous connective tissue found throughout your body, more specifically the fascia. World-renowned anatomist and Align Podcast regular Gil Hedley has described fascia as "a three-dimensional network that gives us our shape and allows us to sense the world around us."

For a long time, our eyes were thought to be the richest sensory organ, but recent research has deemed fascia to be the king of sensation, boasting more than 100 million sensory nerve endings. Your body can actually react and move in response to stimulus before sending the message all the way to the brain and back, which would be too slow to allow you to react when you suddenly slip on ice or step off a curb unknowingly. In fact, fascial pioneer

Robert Schleip has demonstrated that fascia contains myofibroblasts, which allow smooth-muscle-like contraction to occur.[1] This highly intelligent tissue is what anatomists used to throw away in dissection and refer to as the "packing peanuts" of the body.

Our brains are continually receiving an immense amount of information through the connective tissue, which is constantly forming a body schema of where your parts are in space. These sensory organs can determine the temperature of your surroundings, detect sound, send signals of pain to indicate danger or potential tissue damage, and are on the ready to relax, contract, or whatever needs to be done to keep that precious body of yours safe.[2] Every stimulus is like a lesson for your nervous system. "Bad things are not the worst things that can happen to us. NOTHING is the worst thing that can happen to us," said American novelist Richard Bach. Your nervous system grows and thrives on adaptation in the form of movement variation (including moving your senses). For this reason, a sedentary lifestyle or *nothing* at all is one of the worst things that can happen to the human organism.

PLUGGING BACK INTO THE GRID

Think of your body as an electrical grid. If you've ever flown in a plane over a city at night, you saw some homes or parts of the town lit up and others shrouded in darkness. The dark spots are locations of inactivity or perhaps even abandonment; we have similar "dark spots" in our bodies. Your movement awareness is what lights those dark spots through activity and introspection; if you're having issues with balance, pain, or weakness in certain areas of your body, it may be because you need to reconnect those areas of your body to the power grid.

In order to get the lights back on in the dark sectors of town, we need to cultivate communication between everyone involved. The body may be getting bombarded by signals of distress due to chronic tissue dehydration, compression from imbalanced postural patterns, a lack of regular restorative movement, or a nervous system stuck in a "fight, flight, or freeze" state due to mental, emotional, and/or environmental signals. Upon beginning this process, your brain will likely have a lot of static to deal with. It will take some doing to light the place back up, but it can be done with awareness of some simple fundamentals and a splash of intention.

CHANGING YOUR SHAPE

I've heard it said that our muscles are slaves to our posture. You could also say they're both slaves to the nervous system. The reality is these perspectives are all different ways of chopping up a continuous system; you cannot affect any part of your organism without impacting the whole in the very same moment. The good news, though, is that you have the power to impact all the systems via shifting your shape as though you're chiseling a living sculpture. This is what Ida Rolf was referring to when she said, "We work with the body because it's what we can get our hands on." Perhaps *the* superpower of humans is our immense capacity for adaptation. For the most part, your environment is like an artist continually shaping your malleable muscles, bones, and connective tissue.

Literally every physical (and emotional) aspect of your day—your car seat, chairs, walking paths, shoes, clothing, bike, screens, job, and anything else you come in contact with—leaves a subtle imprint, just like a potter's hands pressing into clay. This is what makes the modern mold of chair hunching and screen staring so dangerous: Our bodies literally become *molded* to these shapes.

In science speak, this is referred to as Davis's law, which states your soft tissue re-forms itself based on the imposed demands of your life. With time, these subtle imprints become deep divots and possibly ruts that require work, intention, and know-how to rebalance and restore. That's the good news: You *can* undo the forward head posture, rolled forward shoulders, hunched-over spine, imbalanced pelvis, collapsed knees, and flat feet that our modern environments have crafted so many of our bodies to become. These are all directly tied to the emotional states of feeling "depressed" or "down," but you can rise above them and begin reshaping into an upright, flexible, strong, aligned version of yourself. As you do so, your mood will change for the better, too.

TENDING TO THE GARDEN

Your connective tissue could be likened to fast-growing bushes; our movement is the act of pruning, maintaining, and structuring the growth, like training the branches of a tree to fit your vision. In fact, it's been shown that when an acupuncture needle penetrates the skin, collagen fibers coil around the needle literally like a living vine wrapping around a lattice. There's a whole moving world inside of you, and you're the orchestrator of the show based on how you inhabit your body (a lot of responsibility, I know). If you don't regularly tend to your internal bushes (connective tissue), they begin to grow out of control and agglutinate (firmly stick together to form a mass) into unresponsive, dense, dehydrated tissue.

This is literally happening right now as you read this. Take a quick scan of your body—is there anything that you want to move? Those signals you feel to twist, turn, stretch, stand up, squat, etc., are all built-in mechanisms (for a healthy person) telling you where to trim next.

An aligned body has all its parts in order to allow fluids to circulate, tissues to heal, and dis-ease to resolve like organizing the pipes within a town's sewage and irrigation systems to remove stagnation and permit growth. Andrew Taylor Still, founder of osteopathy, pioneered many of these ideas. He wrote in his book *Philosophy of Osteopathy*, "The osteopath seeks first physiological perfection of form, by normally adjusting the osseous framework, so that all arteries may deliver blood to nourish and construct all parts. Also, that the veins may carry away all impurities, dependent upon them for renovation. Also, that the nerves of all classes may be free and unobstructed while applying the powers of life and motion to all divisions, and the whole system of nature's laboratory."[3]

This idea is a core foundational principle to grasp as we begin this journey together. As you begin reconnecting different parts of your body to the power grid through daily postural awareness, your body can grow healthier with time instead of giving in to the commonly accepted belief of gradual collapse. Each day is a choice to take an active role in aligning and restoring your structure; the alternative is chaos.

INTERNAL INTELLIGENCE

The basic principles outlined below are sculpting tools to take back control of your form. Each one is powerful and, like any tool, becomes more potent as you learn to wield it correctly. The most powerful tool you have at your disposal is your own internal intelligence—the awareness of your own body and the meaning of its many messages. The way to cultivate control of the happenings within your body is to simply begin paying attention.

One form of this is awareness is referred to as "interoception," which loosely translates to your perception of the internal state of your body, such as organ function. In *The Body Keeps the Score*, Bessel van der Kolk describes it as our awareness of our inner body–based feelings. He suggests that with greater awareness, we have greater potential to gain control of our lives and that knowing *what* we feel is the first step to knowing *why* we feel that way.[4] Cultivating awareness of your own internal landscape is like spending time in the metaphoric garden mentioned above, learning what's planted where and how to tend to the various flora and fauna inhabiting the space. In literal terms, this includes mindfulness, breath work, self-care techniques, manual therapy, and movement practice to develop your body's internal senses.

Then we have "neuroception," a term coined by the distinguished university professor Dr. Stephen Porges. In his book *The Polyvagal Theory*, he defines neuroception as "how neural circuits distinguish whether situations or people are safe, dangerous or life threatening." At a sub-cognitive level, we are continually making judgments about our surroundings to determine whether we should fight, flee, freeze, or socially engage with the world around us. The coming chapters offer tools on how to successfully navigate this neurophysiological ladder. Side note: I think this may have been what Rumi was referring to when he said, "The moment you entered this world, a ladder was placed in front of you that you might transcend."

Finally, there is "proprioception," your sense of the relative position of your own body parts in space, and the strength of effort employed in movement. Such introspective awareness is a sixth sense and a missing link in the healthcare of modern humans, leading to greater risk of injury, diminished cognitive function, and a loss of confidence in one's ability to feel powerful and confident in their own mind and body. This book is about turning your sixth sense back on!

ALIGNMENT TOOLS

Throughout the rest of the book, I'm going to share with you the exercises, practices, and tools you can use to develop internal intelligence and craft your body based on its individual needs. I'm going to introduce you to some fundamental movement practices and lifestyle shifts to boost your productivity, creativity, and overall energy levels. Before we begin, there are some simple self-care tools that I've found immensely helpful over the years. There's no absolute need to have any of them to take advantage of the advice in this book. That being said, they're all affordable and game changers for your quality of movement.

Yoga Block

This is exactly what it sounds like, a rectangular block made of cork, wood, or foam typically acting as a support by raising the ground in specific areas to assist in bringing your body into better alignment during yoga (or any movement practice, including just sitting on the floor). Blocks are often used to adjust the height of your hips for proper alignment, but their uses stretch far beyond this. Grab a couple of differently sized cushions and blocks—they'll come in handy. If you don't have a block handy, a stack of books will do just fine!

Kettlebell

A kettlebell looks a bit like a cannonball with a handle or a heavy teakettle (hence the name). Kettlebells were used originally several hundred years ago in Russia as counterweights to weigh dry goods on market scales until, like so many amazing inventions, people began to play with them. These little fellas certainly pack a punch for strengthening but also can be used as self-care tools by laying their weight into stuck tissue and using the techniques described in this chapter to rehydrate the area. If you have limited space, a few kettlebells of varying sizes will go a long way for at-home functional movement training. If you don't have a kettlebell handy, you could get away with a few dumbbells.

Pull-Up Bar

This is such an amazing tool to have indoors if you don't have regular access to gym or playground equipment. Grab one for your doorway today, and be sure to carefully follow the installation instructions. If you don't have a pull-up bar nearby, go outside and find a tree branch to hang from. Your neighbors may think you're a bit crazy, but it could also inspire them to save their shoulders and decompress their own spines!

Lacrosse Ball

My travel self-care bag is real simple: a ball and a band. They're both super light, fit easily in a carry-on bag, and serve lots of different purposes. Avoid getting lots of specialized equipment and stick to the basics, as simple tools are the most dependable and versatile. Another great option for something a bit softer than a lacrosse ball is a set of Tune Up Fitness Balls from my friend and fascia queen, Jill Miller. If none of these options are available, you can get a lot of good self-care work done with a smooth rock or the edge of a couch.

Foam Roller

For rolling out at home, feel free to get foam rollers in a couple different densities to feel what is best for your tissue. I recommend the Melt Method Rollers for a softer option made by my other friend and fascial superhero, Sue Hitzmann. For travel, I recommend using a thick water bottle as a foam roller (Mobot is a solid option).

Align Band

My most frequently used tool with clients over the years has been a resistance band for both home and travel use to mobilize tissues and reorganize joints. The issue for clients using resistance bands for mobility is they typically don't have a good place to attach the band—that's why the Align Band includes a door anchor inside the travel case so you can hang it from any hotel, car, or closet door. Think of the resistance band as the sculptor's chisel and the various techniques below as techniques for effectively reshaping your body. You can get a free complete video guide on how to effectively use resistance bands for self-care and functional movement at www.alignband.com.

Throughout the book, I'll focus on how you can use the Align Band to steadily realign your body, mobilize your joints, and rehydrate your connective tissue.

FUNDAMENTAL MOBILITY TECHNIQUES

You can utilize the techniques below along with the self-care tools mentioned above with the help of a friend or by yourself. The techniques are universal for any body and are what I've most consistently used in my manual therapy practice for the last decade to help clients of all levels achieve their structural goals.

Contract-Relax

It's very simple: As you're stretching the desired muscle group, take your joint toward its comfortable end range of motion and contract with anywhere from 20 percent to 90 percent maximal tension for approximately five seconds. Then breathe out, release the contraction, and watch yourself stretch a bit further into the motion as if by magic. This technique takes advantage of the nervous system's spinal cord reflexes that inhibit/relax your muscle tone and act as a great way to pump fluid into the cells of the targeted area for better tissue hydration.

The contraction activates your stretch reflex (which attempts to protect by shortening your muscles in danger) to temporarily take a vacation while you inch out new ranges of motion. This magical process is in part attributed to the Renshaw cells in the spinal cord sending the signal back to the muscle, explaining to it that your muscles are contracting already, and the stretch reflex can back off from contracting even more to protect you. You can use this technique anywhere you find yourself with some shortened muscles and watch your body literally begin to re-form before your eyes.

Pin and Stretch

This technique is one the most effective ways to unglue matted connective tissue and bring new hydration into previously dried-up tissues. Your body has 640-odd muscles (varying depending on the person) that work most effectively when they're differentiated from each other and not all bound up from being squashed together with chronic chair sitting. Think of your movement like playing a piano. If you slam your hands down on all the keys at the same time, you will have earsplitting cacophony. That's what it's like for your body when the tissue is all stuck together in gunked-up slabs, instead of possessing the capacity to slide freely. This is what we're achieving with these techniques— helping once sliding surfaces to slide again. Viva the sliding surface revolution!

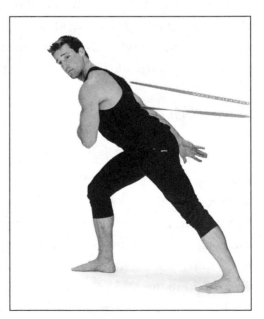

The Pin and Stretch technique is just like it sounds: You'll pin the targeted spot you'd like to work with down by pressing your weight into the band or whatever self-care tool you're using. Once the tissue is "pinned," you begin stretching by moving your joint in such a way to lengthen the targeted area. In the example to the right, the band is pinning down the trapezius muscles and you turn your neck to the opposite direction to create a pull through the connective tissue all the way down the neck and shoulder. Remember to focus on your ease of breath and try to make your exhalation a couple of seconds longer than your inhalation to help calm the nervous system and create more length and tissue relaxation. Breathe through your nose to amplify the positive effects.

Passive Mobility

I find working passively—meaning not adding active movement or contraction to the technique—to be helpful with people whose nervous systems are more tense or high-strung to begin with. You could use passive stretching with or without any self-care tools. An example of this would be a forward fold in yoga, in which you just relax and let your body fold while you breathe into the body parts you would like to target. You could also use the Align Band to assist in passive mobilizations by simply passing the band around the joint you are mobilizing. In the forward fold

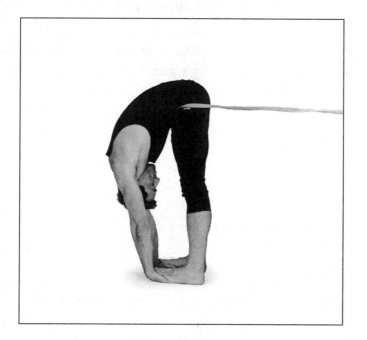

example, you'd wrap the band around your abdomen and fold over it. Once again, breathe into the band and use it as a feedback mechanism to relax your gut and lengthen the spine. In this particular position, you can place your hands under your feet for a deeper stretch and a little hand decompression as well. Enjoy!

Active Mobility

If *passive* mobility means you're not engaging muscles while lengthening them during a stretch, *active* means you are (you're flabbergasted, I'm sure). This is a great way to create more control and intelligence in a joint instead of merely expanding range of motion without movement competence in the position, which could actually increase likelihood of injury. Dr. Andreo Spina of Functional Anatomy Seminars refers to this as "owning your range of motion." Here's what you do: While going through any of the mobility techniques mentioned in this book, actively contract the muscles you are lengthening against the resistance of the stretch. If you get to a point in the mobilization that you can't actively contract the targeted muscles while stretching, you've reached the limit of your active mobilization. You can begin with contracting against the stretch with around 50 percent strength and slowly ramp it up to 90 percent as it feels safe for you. Take three to five slow, deep breaths through your nose while engaging in these end ranges of motion and, with control, slowly return the joint back to its original position. Repeat two to three times or as feels helpful. Avoid the "no pain, no gain" mantra in any form of mobility work—it should feel good.

Visualization

"Where there is no vision, the people perish."
—*Proverbs 29:18*

It's easy to dismiss something like visualization as being too "woo woo," but you'll hear time and time again of elite athletes describing the deep level of detail they go into pre-competition when visualizing exactly what they're about to perform. Could there be something more to this than just psyching themselves up before an event? Could they literally be programming their muscles to function the way they would need to for the live situation they're painting in the mind? Science says we can actually strengthen our muscles just by focusing our minds on a specific movement with no visible action at all. Yogis have been exploring this for years, placing their awareness into specific parts of the body during asana practice or meditation. Our minds and bodies have evolved together, and it appears there is less of a separation (if any at all) than most would expect. It is apparent you can induce change in your tissues by merely placing your mind into the targeted areas and visualizing your intended effects.

A study from Ohio University demonstrated this by recruiting twenty-nine volunteers and wrapping their wrists in surgical casts for a total of four weeks, asking half of them to think about exercising their immobilized wrists for eleven minutes a day, five days a week. They sat totally still and focused on mentally flexing their wrists during the mental training sessions. After the casts were removed, the subjects who visualized wrist exercises had double the wrist strength of those who had done nothing at all![5]

A team at the University of Washington showed imaginary exercise to activate the same brain areas as those of actual movement-based exercise, and the Cleveland Clinic conducted a study showing that imaginary finger exercises strengthen finger muscles by 35 percent.[6] It is becoming more and more abundantly clear that the mind is perhaps *the* most powerful tool in creating not just tissue change but change in the shape of your life. William James said, "The greatest discovery of my generation is people can alter their lives by altering their states of mind." I would venture to say the greatest discovery of my career is that people can change the tonicity of their connective tissues and nervous system function by altering their states of mind and reciprocally alter their state via affecting the body. The mind and body are inextricably linked, like two sides of the same coin. It's a little wordy, I know, but you get the point.

Whether you're trying to mobilize a stuck joint, rehydrate gunky tissue, or activate inhibited muscles, visualize exactly what you'd like to achieve within your body. You could visualize cool ocean water pouring into the targeted tissue and each breath as the tide pulling fluid in and out, washing out the old stagnant fluid and refreshing with crystal clear water. If you want to activate an area, you could imagine electricity moving into the targeted muscle groups as you're activating them. Then every time you initiate a contraction, it's like a lightning bolt charging the tissue up. Do whatever works for you and play with visualizing more things in your life in general, as it's more powerful than you may think.

The tools and movements in this chapter are some of the fundamentals of movement that can help get you in touch with your body. Try them out, see what feels good, pay attention to what feels uncomfortable, and see what your body begins to respond to. Throughout the rest of the book, I'll be sharing with you specific exercises and techniques for releasing pain and building stability. You can think of floor sitting, hip hinging, and the other movement practices in this book as investing in a retirement plan. Every time you hang, for example, it's like dropping a dollar into your long-term health fund. The added benefit of this fund is you start profiting from it immediately! Your health will be the most important thing to you at some point in your life, even if it isn't at this moment. Before you hit a crisis point, you can start taking better care of yourself right now. Visualize yourself literally dropping money into your strength, flexibility, and overall vitality fund every time you activate any of the practices discussed in the book, and watch your portfolio grow. Eventually, your metaphoric money is working for you even while you sleep, and your health dividends grow by the manner in which you *live*.

Alignment Assignment

Start developing your interoceptive abilities with this simple exercise. Sit in a comfortable position and set a timer for one minute. Start the timer and count how many of your own heartbeats you can sense during the minute. Then, do it again by taking your pulse from either your neck or wrist and see how close the two counts are. With practice, you will find that the numbers begin getting closer and closer. This is a powerful tool to center and calm yourself anytime you feel a bit stressed!

PART II

5 DAILY MOVEMENTS TO ALIGN YOURSELF

CHAPTER 4

Floor Sitting: Your Foundation for Self-Care

"You can't solve a problem with the same thought process that started the problem."

—*Albert Einstein*

The first of the 5 Daily Movements we're going to explore might be surprising: floor sitting. It's easy to vilify sitting as the scourge to your health, but in reality sitting is just another form of movement. The way you sit and the variety of positions you choose are of equal importance (if not more) to the amount of time spent sitting. Let me explain.

Does anyone else find the abundance of chair-sitting-based exercise equipment in gyms a bit redundant, as though we don't practice that position enough in modern culture as it is? Let's paint a quick picture of most people's daily leg and hip use. We bend slightly to roll out of a raised bed, wake up, and walk out to the kitchen where everything is conveniently placed at hip level or above, removing the need to squat or even hip hinge for that matter. Hopefully, at some point you drop a deuce by sitting to about ninety degrees on a raised toilet, then shuffle out to the car, bus, or train to sit in the same posture. Next, it's off to work, where you most likely assume the repetitive position once again, but now in either a prestigious leather chair or whatever crummy butt retainer is provided by your employer (or perhaps you're progressive and stand in place while working).

Come clocking out time, it's back to the car seat again, then maybe you go to the gym where you likely spend at least some of your time sitting on a bike, rowing device, or a few seated weight machines. Next you take your sweaty self back to your car seat, before heading home to fall back into a chair at your dining room table for dinner. To finish the day, you retreat to the couch to decompress and watch some well-deserved Netflix. Did you notice anything missing here? How about any activity that would require you to demonstrate range of motion below hip level or above shoulder level? These missing movements serve as the foundation for the health and vitality of modern human beings, and it's far easier to restore their function than you might think.

This tale of repetitive strain reminds me of the story of Amar Bharati, a Sadhu man who has held his right arm up over his head as a tribute to Shiva for more than forty years. At this point, his arm is atrophied with tissues dehydrated and stiffened into a statuesque position, like a human flagpole saluting to God. It sounds absolutely insane for a person to go through the pain of allowing their perfectly healthy tissues to become stiff and rigid to the point of losing function, but I would venture to suggest many people in Western culture are going through a similar process within their ankles, hips, shoulders, and spines. Think about it: Most of us have spent the majority of our waking lives hunched over on chairs with our hips flexed to ninety degrees, but instead of sacrificing joint function in the name of God, we're doing it in the name of Google.

TEST YOURSELF

I've always been curious at what point exactly in a person's life one loses the physical sense of youth. A distinguishing factor I see among seemingly *old* people is an inability to comfortably get down and up from the ground to play with a dog, or child, or just sit on the grass in a park. In fact, there was an interesting study published in the *European Journal of Preventive Cardiology* that featured a useful test I'd like you to take.

It's aptly referred to as the sitting-rising test: You start from a standing position and attempt to smoothly sit all the way to the ground using the least number of contact points with the ground possible other than your feet and butt. From there, you fold into a cross-legged position, and then do the same with standing back up. If you can go through this whole movement sequence smoothly with no extra contact points, you score a perfect ten. For each contact point, such as using a hand or knee for support on the way up or down, deduct one point. If you wobble at any moment, deduct a half-point from your score. According to research, middle-aged and elderly people (age fifty-one to eighty) who needed to use both hands and knees to get up and down, averaging the lowest scores (0–3), were almost six times more likely to die during the 6.3-year span of the study compared to those who scored 8–10 points!

One of the study co-authors, Claudio Gil Soares de Araújo, a professor at Gama Filho University in Rio de Janeiro, suggested this to be an excellent test to indicate a person's flexibility, balance, and motor coordination. He said, "Moving, for the average person, especially those who are older, and the ability to rise from the floor is very much relevant for autonomy."[1] This is a serious conversation for the elderly of Western culture, as one in four people age sixty-five–plus fall each year, and the total cost of the injuries was $50 billion in 2015.[2] It's also worth mentioning the 1.8 million total hip and knee replacement surgeries performed worldwide each year could be significantly ameliorated with a daily dose of mobility via more floor time.

The good news is such immobility is preventable and reversible. This simple movement sequence of regularly moving up and down from the ground is a testament to a person's flexibility, strength, balance, and motor coordination. These are primary factors of vitality, and the floor is the training ground to cultivate them.

FUNDAMENTAL PATTERNS ARE CHILD'S PLAY

Time spent on the ground acts as a natural tuning mechanism for your whole body (if you follow the guidelines of the positions mentioned later in the chapter). I gathered the language of tuning the body through resting positions of repose from the book *Muscles and Meridians* by Phillip Beach. He brings up the powerful point that all cultures, of all ages, until recently spent all or most of their resting time and much of their working time on the ground. The stress of the day can be taxing on the body, and time spent on the ground naturally restores your function by massaging your tissues, mobilizing your joints, and passively retuning the nervous system via a handful of fundamental movement patterns that Beach refers to as "archetypal postures of repose." Some of these positions include kneeling, squatting, toe sitting, crossing your legs, and simply lying down (on flat ground instead of mushing into a couch all the time).

A deep squat position has been the resting position for most of earth's populace for millennia. The cultures still regularly using these archetypal postures of repose in their daily lives exhibit minimal incidence of fall risk and/or osteoarthritis in the hips and knees. There are many neurological benefits to these floor-based movement patterns too, including memory consolidation, brain hemisphere integration, and overall neural development. These core movements and resting positions act as natural physical tuning mechanisms to reorganize our body parts after a long day of work. Beach says:

> It's proposed that these "archetypal postures of repose" are a self-tuning mechanism for a complex musculoskeletal system. Removing self-corrective modes is asking for trouble. We need floor sitting to preserve our biomechanical tune that is the profound interaction of many muscles and joints that summate to produce floor postures that provide us with ease and rest.[3]

We've been widely taught that the way to get a healthy body is to work harder; if you're unsatisfied with your progress, it's likely due to a lack of grinding at the gym. But in reality, your rest practice is equally as valuable as your active movement practice or *exercise*: They're two sides of the same coin. This is a primary missing link in our present healthcare and "fitness" model. We're leaving an immense amount of restorative time on the table (or chair/couch, in this case), and it's causing us pain.

Want to reverse it? Simply adding some floor time today is just what you need to move the needle on beginning the process of harmonizing your body.

You will feel beneficial effects within minutes, such as hip and ankle mobility along with spinal decompression, from the positions mentioned below. A friendly warning: Once you start incorporating more floor time into your day and feel the short- and long-term beneficial effects, it will be very uncomfortable to go back to a high quantity of chair sitting.

IN DWELLING, LIVE CLOSE TO THE GROUND

I have a not-so-secret plan to bring sexy back to spending more time on the ground each and every day. Ancient Chinese philosopher Lao-tzu would be with me on this; he once said, "In dwelling, live close to the ground. In thinking, keep to the simple." We've come up with some pretty clever contraptions to get chiseled abs, broad shoulders, or an attractive booty, but along the way we've missed the simplicity of where our bodies and minds have evolved from for millions of years: the ground.

Generally speaking, the more complex the "fitness" apparatus, the less intelligent the body needs to be in order to use it. Our brain is brilliant at conserving energy, and if you outsource the need to stabilize, balance, or use a range of motion to a machine, the muscles and neural connections innervated to perform those actions begin to atrophy and wither away. You could certainly put the chair into this category of body-dumbing apparatus: By removing the regular need to squat below the height of your seated platform, you begin to lose the ability to do so. You were easily able to get into and sustain an "ass to grass" squat at one point in your life and it's still re-attainable. The ground is a noble and gradual teacher with the power to heal your joints and recover ranges of motion you thought had been lost.

Our joints are self-healing systems so long as we offer them the basic raw materials to repair. These materials include proper nutrition, cycles of lightness and dark, water, grounding, and regular exploration of full ranges of motion in order to circulate fluids and send signals at the cellular level to strengthen all the nooks and crannies of each joint and its surrounding tissue.

Create a designated floor-sitting area in your home. Get yourself a comfy rug or thick floor covering, lots of comfy ground cushions, and ideally make it somewhere that gets lots of natural light. Make it comfortable, fun, and colorful: You'll notice your children, pets, and yourself drawn to this area if you do it right. I'm actually lying on my belly in a sphinx-like yoga position—with a pillow under my pelvis to support my low back and my computer in front of me—as I'm writing this very sentence.

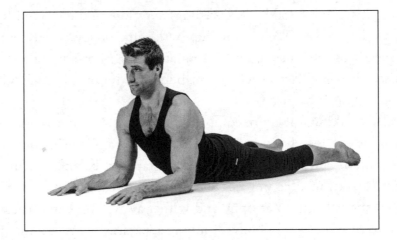

YOU KNEAD MORE FLOOR TIME

There's a fancy word for the cellular response to movement: "mechanotrans-duction," which refers to the process through which cells sense and respond to mechanical stimuli by converting them to biochemical signals that elicit specific responses (a mouthful, I know).[4] You can think of this process as a language translation device; your movement is a language, and your cells translate each individual "word" or movement into a chemical signal that tells your body what to do next.

Your cells respond optimally to being moved around in different directions, similar to the way a pizza maker throws dough for a pie. She needs to massage the dough in a variety of angles to ensure that it forms the soft, stretchy texture that makes great pizza crust. Not working the dough enough results in a brittle, tough consistency that is hard to enjoy. This dough-stretch analogy illustrates what takes place in the physical journey of squatting or lunging all the way to the floor, sitting in a variety of positions as you're massaging your hips on a comfy rug or a floor cushion (exactly what you're *not* doing with the deskbound lifestyle modernity has adopted). Not only is the simple act of spending more time on the ground both healing and strengthening, but it also creates more opportunities to practice the invaluable movement patterns of getting up from the ground to use the bathroom, grab a drink, or answer a phone call. Then you go back down to start it all over again (a lot like what you'd pay a personal trainer $100 an hour to tell you to do at a gym—what a coincidence!).

This full range of up and down from the ground motion serves to rehydrate your hips, strengthen your legs, and re-circulate stagnant fluid from your lower body. Plus, the abdominal pressure created from squatting even acts as a gut massage. John F. Kennedy said, "The time to fix the roof is when the sun is shining." I would add that the time to strengthen your hips is while you still have the ability to do so. Regular exploration of the space between your hips and feet age-proofs your body, so you never have to deal with the dreaded "I've fallen and I can't get up" moment. The kindest thing you can do for your parents, grandparents, and yourself is encourage everyone to spend time each day on the ground. It will pay back hugely in the form of flexibility, strength, balance, coordination, and autonomy for the rest of your life.

THE CIRCULATION EQUATION

Your lymphatic fluid is a crucial component of your immune health and it is dependent on your movement to circulate. Chronic chair sitting turns your lower body into a lymphatic crockpot stewing away while you work. If you've ever rolled an ankle, you likely heard the advice to lie down and prop your feet up to assist in circulating blood back to the heart. The same idea applies to floor sitting—you can more efficiently pump your blood by reducing the vertical height your heart is away from your feet compared to chair sitting.

This brings us to the topic of standing desks, which are certainly a step in the right direction, but only get us part of the way down the road to resolving the musculoskeletal issues of modernity. Excessive standing has its own list of problems. The healthiest (that's right, I'm intentionally using a superlative) positions for spending a lot of time in are on the ground. We're primordially coded to these fundamental positions, and they're a powerful antidote to the tightness and pain many people experience today. If you are deskbound, I have some recommendations for how to adjust the configuration of your workspace and change the patterns of your workday later in the book (see Chapter 11).

FLOOR SITTING AS SPIRITUAL PRACTICE

Americans spent $16.5 billion in 2013 on treating osteoarthritis (OA), a debilitating and painful condition affecting more than 30 million adults in the United States. You'd think with all of our amazing technology and high quality of living we would be ameliorating any pesky joint issues of the past. But in fact, developing countries such as those in North Africa, the eastern Mediterranean, and Southeast Asia exhibit the lowest incidence of OA.[5] They have half the rate of OA of the knee and almost no OA of the hip, compared to the countries with higher prevalence of such joint issues.

I've spent extended periods of time in all of these places and observed specific things consistently within their lifestyles that are undoubtedly primary contributors to their joint health. You guessed it: They all spend more time on the ground—during food preparation, meals, and social time.

I still remember the loudspeakers blaring through the streets of Marrakech, Morocco (North Africa), reminding people to pray. Prayer, in Islam, is not just a moment of spiritual connection; it is also a physical ritual in which believers take their bodies through archetypal postures of repose and renewal multiple times per day. Religion aside, regular stretching is an immensely powerful healthcare practice that if applied to Western culture would be an absolute game changer for ankle, knee, hip, spine, and mental health. Think about the implications. Daily calls to prayer encourage people to get up with the sun (a part of the Aligned Morning), take a walk to the nearest mosque or place of prayer (Walking), meditate regularly (Mindfulness), squat down to the ground into a kneeling position (Hip Hinging and Floor Sitting), and then reach their arms over their head while on the floor (Hanging). While they're on the ground, they say a prayer in a rhythmic way (Sound) all the while connecting with community (Touch) at least five times per day!

A sequence of movement such as this is literally a foundation of your evolution as a hominid. These movements are ingrained in your system as a natural strengthening, lengthening, and overall tuning mechanism for your ankles, knees, hips, and spine, like a key in an evolutionary lock. Not to mention that ground sitting facilitates the circulation of lymphatic fluids via the compression of your tissues from various contact points with the ground and the up-and-down movement that's inevitable each time you need to change locations.

Perhaps an original foundation of many religious dogmas is assisting people to connect with their own minds and bodies, as we see with the Muslim religion. Following all five daily movements of this book each day is a means to stay connected to source (whatever that means to you). The simple act of getting down and up off the ground on a regular basis is downright biblical, as in kneeling or prostrating oneself in prayer. Along with walking, this is one of the most nurturing full-body exercises we can do. Our Westernized model has removed us from the floor and inadvertently made it a symbol of childishness, low economic status, and bad hygiene.

We seek to seize the highest place, whether it's the head of the boardroom table, the driver's seat of a fancy SUV, or some other obscure seat we think connotes power and influence. Perhaps this physical act of bending down low is an aspect of what is meant in Luke 14:10–11, when Jesus told his disciples, "When you are invited, take the lowest place, so that when your host comes, he will say to you, 'Friend, move up to a better place.' Then you will be honored in the presence of all your fellow guests. For everyone who exalts himself will be humbled, and he who humbles himself will be exalted."

BURN FAT AND STAY BLUE

"Men are born soft and supple; dead they are stiff and hard.
Plants are born tender and pliant; dead, they are brittle and dry.
Thus whoever is stiff and inflexible is a disciple of death.
Whoever is soft and yielding is a disciple of life."

—the *I Ching*

People raised in the Blue Zones (a term popularized by author Dan Buettner for locations with a high percentage of centenarians) of the world are certainly movers, but generally don't care much about traditional gym exercise. Rather, their lifestyle is such that movement is baked into each day: getting down on the ground in kneeling, squatting, and lunging positions to tend to a garden, walking to town to buy groceries, easy access to impromptu games of soccer (or football, as it's known in the rest of the world outside of good ole 'Merica) with their children in the street or village square. Exercise is an abstract waste of energy from much of the world's perspective.

In fact, the sense of accomplishment exercising cultures feel post-workout can even create an "illusory invulnerability," a term coined by a Chinese research team.

When taking a health supplement or doing a hard workout, people often tend to make worse decisions because they've feel they earned it. A blow-out training session helps reduce fidgety restlessness, but those regular micro-movements referred to as fidgeting serve as a mini-workout distributed throughout the whole day, which turns out to be optimal for your health! Joan Vernikos, former director of life sciences at NASA, spent more than forty years observing the health of astronauts in space and found regular movement distributed throughout the day to be more effective at preventing the deleterious effects of space travel than a large dose of exercise followed by a sedentary workday (a principle at the heart of her 2011 book *Sitting Kills, Moving Heals*).

James Levine, inactivity researcher at the Mayo Clinic in Rochester, Minnesota, has extensively studied the effects of non-exercise activity thermogenesis (NEAT) on the health and specifically weight gain of humans. NEAT is essentially the various movements you do during the day you may not think of as exercise, per se, but that are in fact burning calories and, more importantly for the sake of this book, toning, tuning, and aligning your various body parts with one another. Examples of how to include more NEAT (other than more time on the ground) could include cleaning your house, cooking, doing yard work, helping a friend move, etc.[6]

It's about to get even stranger: Your mere awareness of the health benefits associated with seemingly mundane movements such as these can create observable physiological change compared to mindlessly performing the tasks. In a past Align Podcast episode, Harvard psychologist Ellen Langer discussed how she demonstrated this in a study involving eighty-four hotel maids, in which she told only forty-four of them about the various health benefits of their movement while cleaning the rooms.[7] The results were staggering: The maids who were told about the advantages of their regular movement beforehand were able to lower blood pressure, lose weight, and improve body fat and waist-to-hip ratios. It turns out your movement awareness could be more powerful than most any weight loss pill you could ever find and is completely drawback-free! Pretty NEAT, huh? (My apologies for that—it was just too easy.)

This touches on a primary goal of this book: to expand the world's perception of fitness to be the manner in which you inhabit your body in any situation. You can easily move more effectively and intentionally during all of these household or work activities so that your whole life becomes developmental for your mind, body, and movement. The result will be increased flexibility, strength, balance, and mental clarity.

In Levine's research, he found people's NEAT to vary by more than 2,000 calories per day depending on their lifestyle and non-exercise-related movements throughout the day. The extra calories you'll burn each day by making the ground a more hospitable place to spend time has the power not only to maintain your autonomy into old age, avoid troublesome joint issues such as osteoarthritis and hip disease of all sorts, but will also help move the needle with fat loss!

Dr. Levine concludes: "This information collectively demonstrates that there may be a NEAT defect in human obesity and that this effect is underpinned by a profound yet subtle biology. If one is born with the genetic trait to sit, is obesity inevitable? I do not think so, because obesity emerged over the past century and especially the past 20 years, but our genes did not change. Chair-living has proven so enticing that we have forsaken our legs. It is now time to find ways to get us back onto our legs."[8]

POSITIONS OF REPOSE

> "If you know the way broadly you will see it in everything."
> —Miyamoto Musashi, Japanese soldier-artist
> and author of The Book of Five Rings

How has the rest of the world (for thousands of years) rested and/or worked on projects from the ground, you ask? Here are some fundamental floor sitting positions specifically designed to mobilize your joints and bring your whole body back into tune during and after the stress of the day.

Easy Pose (Sukhasana)

The word "Sukhasana" is derived from the Sanskrit word *sukha*, meaning pleasure or comfort, and *asana*, meaning pose. Remember "criss-cross applesauce," Indian pose, or the W sitting position from elementary school, before your hips froze over like Shackleton's Antarctic journey from excessive desk sitting? This tightening is *not* a natural part of becoming an adult; it's a perversion of our structure, a maladaptation from a dysfunctional movement mold.

The cross-legged position is shown to help mobilize tight hips, disengage overly tight hamstring muscles, and assist in reactivating the butt muscles. This may have something to do with why yogis have spent so much time in this position for literally thousands of years (well, not in a row, but you get the point). It also helps relax and expand your breath, calm your nervous system, facilitate better circulation, and make you superficially appear more conscious or woke to people who care about that sort of thing.

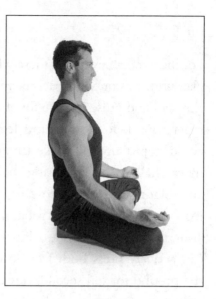

90/90 Position

The name refers to your legs being in ninety-degree angles at both knees and both facing the same direction like two spokes of a pinwheel (a symbol for the sun, well-being, prosperity, and good luck). This position is a great way to mobilize both medial and external rotation of the hip joint. We could alternate between the 90/90 and easy pose throughout our sitting practice, every ten minutes at least.

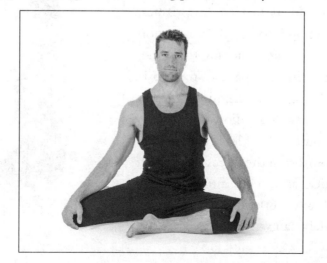

MOVEMENT TIP

For the overachievers out there who would like to make this a more active position, play with raising your back-facing leg up off the ground as high as you comfort-

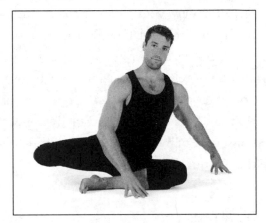

ably can and pulse it there for about ten repetitions before switching legs. You could step it up and make things even more challenging by raising the leg up and rotating the foot up toward the ceiling, creating a medial rotation from your femur (thigh bone). Finally, you can actively press both feet down into the ground for ten seconds, creating an isometric contraction on both sides.

Kneeling (Japanese Style, or Seiza)

This is one of the standard positions you'll see in many martial arts studios around the world. It's a great practice for mobilizing the knee joint and its surrounding tissues, opening the feet up into the plantar-flexion (toe point) position, and stacking the spine. Perhaps this is why in Japanese, this position is referred to as *seiza*, meaning "correct sitting." You can add a pillow or cushion between your butt and ankles if you experience any discomfort in the knees. Start with as much cushion as you need to feel comfortable and slowly work your way down to none if you safely can without experiencing any pain.

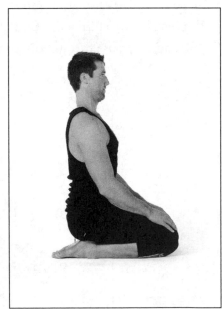

Toe Sit

This position has been one of the most valuable sitting postures to heal my own knees and ankles after years of discomfort. Oftentimes, knee issues are the upstream effect of imbalanced feet; this position is a fantastic check-in on toe and plantar fascia mobility. Your feet have about a zillion possible ranges of motion, and modern shoes act as a huge limiting factor to your foot mobility potential.

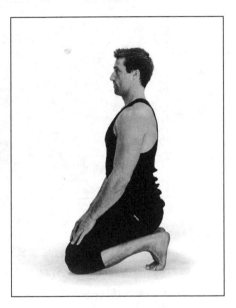

Start from the kneeling position with your knees on a cushion and bring your hands to the ground so you can raise your feet up off the floor. Spread your toes wide and bring them down to the ground as far forward toward your knees as you comfortably can. Once your toes are pressed onto the ground, slowly sit down on your heels (be gentle with this and feel free to place a pillow or cushion between your butt and heels to make it easier). This will likely be uncomfortable to most people at first, but ease your way into it, and remember what the Greek poet Hesiod said, "If you add a little to a little, and do it again, soon that shall be much."

Straddle

An elite gymnast friend recently mentioned to me that she rarely if ever sets aside time to actually stretch. She spends time in this exact position of repose while reading or watching Netflix, and is one of the most stretchy people I know. The straddle position is a standard for any gymnast and is super helpful for opening up those tight calves and hamstrings you hear everyone complaining about. Remember to stay stacked on the front edge of the sit bones (ischial tuberosities) and feel free to stack your butt up on a cushion to be sure you stay on that sweet spot. If you're stacked, this position should feel comfortable. If you can't sit in this position without your pelvis tucking under, raise your butt with cushions until you can. For less stretchy people, this may be a position to build into with time.

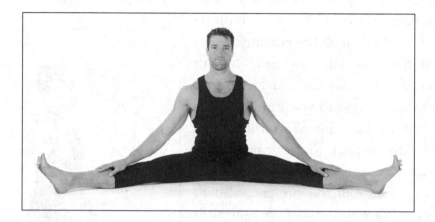

Sphinx

This is the position I am writing most of this book from, if that tells you anything. It's essentially the exact opposite of the position in which we spend most of our school education (physical de-education). We have a long backlog (not especially funny, but a pun nonetheless) of our spines being hunched forward to unwind, and this is a great option to start restructuring the old imbalances. Remember to keep the shoulders down away from the ears and try to focus the extension on the thoracic spine (middle back) instead of the lumbar spine (lower back).

Side-Lying

A beautiful option to open up the side of your body and get into all those gunky nooks and crannies that inevitably build up in the ribs. Try to spend a balanced amount of time on each side, and once again, focus the curve on the thoracic spine instead of the lumbar spine. While side-lying, maintain length through the spine and occasionally press your elbow into the ground to create more length around the neck and shoulder girdle (the tendency will be for your shoulder to collapse up into your neck). Remember to breathe into the areas of tightness.

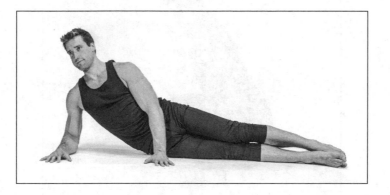

ALIGN YOURSELF

Try this technique to assist in opening your knees and hips to help initiate your joints to more floor time.

Chair Pose (Knee Distraction with Band): Adjust the Align Band to approximately knee height and step both legs through the middle with your body facing the wall. Pass the band behind your knees and step backward to create a pulling tension on the back of your knees. Raise your arms in front of you or overhead depending on your mobility and begin hinging your hips back as though you're sitting into a low chair. Take three full breaths from this low position and with control slowly raise back to standing. Try this technique two to three times to start your day or to create some space in your knees and hips before you sit on the ground.

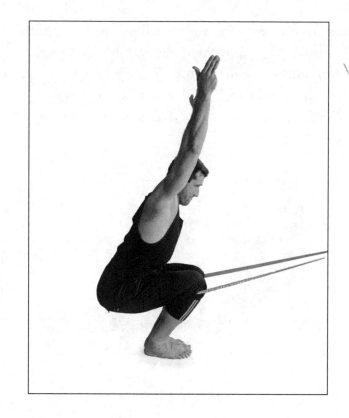

Alignment Assignment

Each day for the next thirty days, devote *at least* thirty minutes to "floor culture." Spend some time on the floor in whatever fashion fits your fancy. You could read, watch TV, check emails, or anything of the sort. (Remember to make the ground comfortable with rugs and cushions). As a general rule: Raise the height of your hips above your knees while sitting so that if you placed a ball on your thigh, it would roll down toward your knees. This will stack your spine to make floor sitting more therapeutic and pleasant over greater amounts of time.

CHAPTER 5

Nasal Breathing: Tuning Your Engine

"Mind is the king of the senses; breath is the king of the mind; and the nerves are the king of the breath."

—Iyengar

The typical adult human takes anywhere from 14,000 to 20,000 breaths a day. But be honest now: When was the last time you thought about even one of these? As breathing is so elemental and could be considered an autonomous action (the body just takes care of it because if you don't breathe, you can't live), we usually don't give it a second thought. And most of the time not even a first one.

That is until we have to. Have you ever been out for a run or done an intense new workout and been left gasping for breath? Do you or does someone you know struggle with asthma that sometimes makes the breath forced or wheezy? Have you ever taken a trip to Colorado or another high-altitude part of the planet and felt like you were sucking air through a straw as you struggled up the side of a mountain?

While such situations are acute and typically rare, they do serve as reminders about the precious nature of breath. Once the overexertion, asthma attack, or lack of altitude acclimation passes, we go right back to forgetting about our breathing. In doing so, we're missing out on an opportunity to regulate our physical, cognitive, and emotional state, while improving sleep, busting stress, and quelling anxiety (no pills required). Let's look at how you can start becoming more aware of your breath so you can manipulate it like a sound engineer at a studio mixing desk to feel and perform the way you want to in any situation. We'll also explore how regulating your breath will benefit your posture and help keep you stable during exercise, even when you start to fatigue.

CHOOSE YOUR STATE

In our always-on, constantly connected, overstimulated world, it's all too easy to get stuck in a state of perma-stress in which it's impossible to truly achieve relaxation. And many of the activities we believe are helping us calm down—cruising our social feeds, watching TV, and so on—are actually revving us up. That's one of the reasons so many people turn to pills or alcohol in the evening: an effort to unwind. Apparently it's not working, at least if sleep researchers are to be trusted. The National Institutes of Health believe that between 50 and 70 million American adults are wandering around like characters from *The Walking Dead* because they get inadequate sleep.[1] And a big reason is that people cannot get out of their all-go, all-the-time mind-set.

The quickest, easiest, and most effective way to alter a physical, cognitive, or emotional state is with breathing. You can think of breath as a remote control for your nervous system. So at night if you're stressed or anxious (and let's face it, these days who isn't?), you can breathe your way into a parasympathetic recovery state using nothing more than the most elemental thing you do: focused nasal breathing. Doing so will enable you to turn down the volume in your amygdala and other regions of the brain responsible for kicking you into a watchful, tense state of high alert.

While most of us could do with taking a chill pill more often, there are certain people who don't just find it difficult to relax, but impossible. These include those suffering from post-traumatic stress disorder (PTSD). A recent study by the University of Wisconsin-Madison's Center for Investigating Healthy Minds concluded that soldiers who performed yogic breathing (aka breaths taken through the nose and initiated in the diaphragm—so called "belly breathing") reported lower anxiety and fewer PTSD symptoms.[2] So even if you've tried everything to help you recover from a traumatizing event like a car wreck and nothing has worked, give breath work a shot.

ALIGN YOURSELF

If you're having trouble winding down at night, try this protocol from my good friend and co-founder of the Art of Breath, Brian Mackenzie. Lie down flat on your couch, bed, or floor and spend at least five minutes breathing in through your nose for five seconds, holding your breath for fifteen seconds, and then exhaling through your nose for ten seconds. If you find yourself in a stressful situation during the day, you can utilize the same protocol, or simply focus on slow nasal inhalations and even slower nasal exhalations for a couple of minutes.

BREATHE TO ACHIEVE

"If you know the art of breathing you have the strength, wisdom, and courage of ten tigers."

—*Chinese proverb*

When I was researching this chapter, I came across a picture of the Australian national rugby team training. I saw the players were all wearing something over their mouths. Wondering what the heck they were up to, I read the accompanying story and learned that they were participating in a breath-retraining program that used such tape to encourage nasal-only breathing.

In a past Align Podcast episode, Buteyko breathing method expert Dr. Patrick McKeown, author of *The Oxygen Advantage*, pointed out that in sports (and life, for that matter), athletes often start mouth breathing way before they redline, or do so from the outset. The problem with this is that it signals to the brain that the body should be in a sympathetic fight-or-flight state. This is fine for short events like a 100-meter sprint or long jump or if you have to flee from a lion, but it isn't sustainable for any length of time.

A major disadvantage of breathing through the mouth during physical exercise is that it is inefficient for a number of reasons. Mouth breathing deemphasizes our diaphragm, which is meant to draw air in and out of our lungs, and instead puts the emphasis on other muscles in the chest, neck, and back that aren't qualified for the job. Once these begin to fatigue from all our huffing and puffing, they start sending signals to the nervous system that we're getting worn out and need to slow down or stop. So we do, often much earlier than is necessary.

As humans we spend a large amount of our time upright, sitting, walking, standing, or running. Because of this, the greatest concentration of blood resides in the lower lobes of the lungs. Breathing through the mouth ventilates the upper lobes, and this is especially likely to occur during physical exercise. Mouth breathing with consequent upper-chest breathing is sabotaging our ability to adequately transfer oxygen from the lungs to the blood.

Breathing through the nose adds a resistance to respiration that is two to three times that of the mouth. When we slow down breathing, the breathing rate reduces, and the size of each breath increases. This significantly improves respiratory efficiency as less air is wasted to dead space. In simple terms, of every breath drawn into the body 150 ml of that air doesn't reach the small air sacs in the lungs where oxygen transfer can take place. Instead, this 150 ml of air remains in the nasal cavity, throat, trachea, bronchi, and bronchioles. If one is breathing fast and shallow, a disproportionately large volume of air remains in dead space.

For example, during exercise, if 20 breaths are drawn into the body over one minute and each breath is 500 ml, this equates to a minute volume of 10 liters.

Subtracting 150 ml from each breath shows that 7 liters of air actually reach the lungs for gas exchange to take place. When we slow breathing down to 10 breaths per minute, and increase the size of each breath to 1 liter, the amount of air that actually reaches the lungs is 8.5 liters. In this example, the amount of air drawn into the body is the same, but the amount of air reaching the small air sacs in the lungs increases when breathing is slow and deep. This translates into a 20 percent improved breathing efficiency simply by slowing the respiratory rate. Nasal breathing forces us to do this; otherwise, the feeling of air hunger is too intense when one breathes fast and shallow. By taping the mouth, we're forced to inhale and exhale only through the nose, which prevents this premature fatigue, increasing endurance and sustained power output. And this isn't just applicable to those big, burly Aussie rugby players. You and I can do it to improve our performance, too.

ALIGN YOURSELF

Not ready to bust out the LipSeal Tape (the brand McKeown recommends) or a cheaper alternative like NexCare Sensitive Skin Tape just yet? Then try this handy tip from Brian Mackenzie: Breathe only through your nose during your workouts. Sounds simple enough, right? Sure, until you hop on your rowing machine and try to bust out a few fast intervals and feel like you're going to pass out.

Don't do that! Instead, back off the intensity a bit until you feel like you can maintain the cadence while still breathing nasally. After a few weeks, your body will get wise and you'll be able to start going faster and harder for longer, while still breathing in and out through your nose. Mackenzie recommends using nasal only in your training for three to four weeks to start. After that, you'll be ready to begin incorporating mouth breathing during maximal efforts as a final "gear," as the Art of Breath co-founder Rob Wilson refers to it.

Think of your breathing style to be like shifting gears in the car of your dreams. Most of the time, it's wise to take it easy on the engine and keep the RPMs at a modest level, but every now and again, it's healthy to have an Autobahn visit and open it up. Here's a simple "Gears System" approach to breathing devised by Wilson for when you want to rev up your engine.

Gear one: Consistent inhalation/exhalation through the nose

Gear two: Fast inhalation through the nose and natural exhalation through the nose

Gear three: Fast inhalation/exhalation through the nose

Gear four: Fast inhalation through the nose and natural exhalation through the mouth

Gear five: Consistent inhalation/exhalation through the mouth until you can comfortably shift back down to a lower gear

(Learn more about the Art of Breath on episode 210 of the Align Podcast or at powerspeedendurance.com.)

YOU SNOOZE, YOU WIN

"When life is foggy, path is unclear and mind is dull, remember your breath. It has the power to give you the peace."

—*Amit Ray*

Another context for utilizing mouth taping that might be even more impactful is at bedtime. Even if you commit to only nasal breathing during the day—and, as we just suggested, during all but the most intense of workouts—you might still be mouth breathing at night. Doing so can undo much of your good work during waking hours, reduce both the quantity and quality of your slumber, and leave you feeling groggy and ill-rested in the morning. It can also put you back in a sympathetic state that messes with your neural and cardiovascular systems. So if you're using a sleep and/or heart rate variability monitor or app and are getting crappy numbers, that's probably why.

Regularly performing some daytime exercises to increase your carbon dioxide tolerance—which is actually what prompts us to take the next breath, not oxygen deprivation—is one way to sort out your nighttime breathing. Exercises like those McKeown shares in *The Oxygen Advantage* can also help you stop over-breathing—that is to say taking unnecessarily deep breaths too frequently. One way to test your carbon dioxide tolerance is to take a BOLT (body oxygen level test) score assessment, which you can determine simply:

1. Take a regular inhale and exhale through your nose.
2. Then, time how long you can hold your breath until you need to breathe (your breath when you resume breathing should be similar to how you were breathing before the breath hold).

While this isn't a college entry test like the ACT or SAT, the results are no less important. Scoring less than twenty-five seconds means you are likely to have sub-optimal breathing patterns. These might all be contributing factors to an excessive feeling of breathlessness during physical exercise, congested nose, exercise-induced asthma, increased stress levels, anxiety, panic disorder, premature muscle fatigue, and, in keeping with the theme of this subsection, sleeping well. If you tally twenty-five to forty seconds, you have a decent tolerance to CO2 but may well be undermining this by mouth breathing during the day or at night, or by "over-breathing"—i.e., taking bigger breaths than you need. If you have sub-optimal breathing during the day, you also have sub-optimal breathing during sleep and physical exercise.

So even if you scored higher, you can still benefit from nasally breathing and making each breath a bit more nonchalant and fairly light. Studies show that reducing your breathing rate to between five and six breaths a minute—fewer than the average of ten to fourteen that "stress breathers" typically take—can significantly improve heart rate variability (HRV), which is one indicator that the parasympathetic "rest-and-digest" branch of the autonomic nervous system is in balance with the sympathetic "fight-or-flight" one.[3] This is essential if you're going to get high-quality, restorative sleep. The sweet spot appears to be five to seven breaths.

Try a brief standing breath practice any time you'd like to calm or gather your-self. So many mindfulness and breathing practices are done while lying down or sitting, which doesn't exactly prepare you to integrate them into your upright life. Here's how it goes: Start in an Aligned Standing position (see Chapter 6, page 88) and follow a basic Box-Breathing pattern of four seconds in, four second hold, four seconds out, four second hold, and repeat for ten rounds of nose breathing. While you're breathing, notice the weight of your body resting into the ground and envision a string lightly pulling the back of your head up toward the sky. You may find it helpful to experiment with placing your hands on the sides of your lower ribs or just under your belly button to guide the breath to these areas for a greater calming effect.

NATURE'S ORTHODONTIST

Chronic mouth breathing day after day doesn't just increase stress and anx-iety. It can also take a toll on a structural level. In the book *Jaws* (nope, it's not about sharks), Sandra Kahn and Paul R. Erlich reveal that children who mouth breathe consistently end up with dental deformities and changes in jaw shape. They assert that if kids would nose breathe instead, we wouldn't need a lot of the expensive orthodontics that parents have to shell out for.[4]

How could this be? you may ask. Try breathing from your mouth for a moment and notice the placement of your tongue. Now close your mouth and take a few breaths through the nose. Notice anything different? When you breathe through your nose, your tongue typically rests on the roof of your mouth, acting like a retainer to prevent your teeth from crowding, and your jaw comes forward instead of collapsing back toward your neck (i.e., the dreaded double chin).

Closing your mouth day and night can not only help prevent snoring and help avoid waking up with a dry mouth, but also can boost sleep quality, prevent the body from entering a sympathetic stress state, and literally change the shape of your face! One remedy: Try the method practiced by the Australian rugby team, but in the evening.

ALIGN YOURSELF

Place a task-specific, cut-to-size product like LipSeal Tape or a piece of sensitive tape from a roll (3M, Nexcare, etc.) lengthwise across your lips before bed. Do it twenty to thirty minutes before bed so you can get used to the sensation before attempting to fall asleep. Have a second strip ready by your bedside in case you wake up to use the bathroom and find the first one has fallen off. To further improve your nighttime breathing, you could consider a nasal dilator like Mute or AirMax. Relationship bonus: It might keep you in the good graces of your significant other by stopping your incessant snoring!

Disclaimer: This is another technique I don't expect everyone to try, nor do I think everyone needs it, but I've heard too many success stories not to mention it as an option to improve sleep quality. Talk with your doctor before trying this if you suffer from any medical issues or experience obstructed breathing of any sort.

BREATH AND MOVEMENT, MOVEMENT AND BREATH

One of the first indicators that we're pushing beyond our limits is we begin either holding our breath or stress-breathing through the mouth. Pay attention when you're trying out a new yoga pose, going for a new personal record in the squat, or trying to keep up with a running partner who's much faster—you'll likely catch yourself mouth breathing around the same time that you start to realize that you're focusing on the result more than you are the process itself. In his excellent book *Endure*, Alex Hutchinson highlights a similar issue in endurance athletes. When their breathing becomes ragged and labored, the respiratory muscles start to seize up, signaling to the brain that they're fatigued. This causes what South African physiologist Tim Noakes calls the "central governor" to spring into action, leading to reduced force production and speed. Eventually the body will just be stopped from moving to protect itself.[5]

A third breath-related problem that athletes often encounter is a lack of stability in their trunk. Inefficient breathing can result in excessive breathing rate and volume, and when breathing is reaching its limit, respiration wins over stability of the spine. Breathing trumps what the body considers less important functions. When we mouth breathe, we minimize the role of the diaphragm. This structure doesn't exist in isolation, but is connected to the rib cage, lumbar spine (not to mention the state of your autonomic nervous system), and some of the primary stabilizing muscles like the psoas. So if the diaphragm is compromised, so too are the parts of the torso that it's connected to. If you're doing a dead lift or squat, or just moving your couch over a couple feet and are breathing fast and shallow through your mouth, you're likely to become unstable and start rounding your back. In contrast, taking a deep nasal breath increases intrathoracic pressure, allowing you to brace against a load (think about picking up a heavy box or deadlifting—there are plenty of scenarios in the gym and real life when you need to stay strong and cohesive through your trunk). The diaphragm moves downwards during inhalation, with the chest cavity acting as a balloon to help provide support and stability for the spine and pelvis. Having functional breathing while lifting helps generate optimal intra-abdominal pressure to reduce the risk of undue spinal compression.[6]

Once again, mouth breathing does have its place, such as when you're in fifth gear (max cardiovascular effort) as discussed previously, or if you need to sip in air quickly for extra intra-abdominal pressure. A lack of movement competence—indicated by uncontrolled breath holding and gasping or collapsing in the torso—can create issues, especially if you're an athlete. By correcting your breathing, you're developing an invaluable tool applicable to any sport, greatly decreasing your risk of injury, and increasing your endurance in every aspect of your life.

Luckily, there's a simple way to fix each of the breath-related movement problems we just explored. First, go back to basics with each of the movements you typically perform in the gym and in your sport. Remove weight, reduce speed, and tune into your breathing. If you notice you're holding your breath or mouth breathing, relax and think consciously about nonchalant nasal breathing. This will likely give you greater movement capacity in the position because you will be signaling to your nervous system that you're not under threat and can relax. When you reach a higher level of exertion at which this becomes impossible, still try to keep a certain pattern for your inhales and exhales, rather than letting your breath get away from you.

When you're about to lift something heavy—be it a bar in the gym or one end of a couch that you're helping a buddy move—stabilize your torso by taking a deep nasal breath and bracing your abs before you commence the lift. This creates what's referred to as intrathoracic pressure, which is a ritzy way of saying that you're keeping your trunk organized because of greater pressure in your chest cavity. Then slowly exhale on the way up.

WAKE UP!

There are some situations where you may be looking for a boost instead of all this slow, calm nasal breathing stuff. Your internal physiology has gears as we mentioned previously and it's possible to simulate opening your engine up even if you're not racing to the top of a mountain. So what do we do if we're feeling low on energy and can't seem to get ourselves into gear, particularly if catching a nap is off the table? Drinking enough coffee to kill a small horse is probably your go-to choice, but that's going to make you feel jittery or sick to your stomach. And if you keep riding the caffeine train all day, it'll further screw up your sleep, perpetuating the vicious cycle many of us know entirely too well.

So if not that, then what? Well, you could try breathing differently. I know this might sound nuts, but bear with me. Just as certain kinds of breathing can help you downshift (nasal, slow exhalations, low rate), so too can other sorts (nasal or mouth, fast exhalations, high rate) put you into fifth gear. That's the beauty of breath control—once you have the basics down, you can work backward from your intended outcome to find the pattern, cadence, and kind of breathing you need to either elevate or down-regulate yourself mentally, physically, and emotionally. When you could use a system reset or an extra boost of energy to crush the day, it may be time to temporarily abandon the nasal-only plan, which applies to most situations, and add in some strong mouth breathing, telling your central computer to get up and at 'em.

BREATHING TECHNIQUE

To introduce a pattern interrupt to your nervous system and add some zeal to your day, we're taking a cue from my friend and extreme athlete Wim Hof. Start with thirty "power" breaths with the following pattern: deep inhale, fast half-exhale (from either nose or mouth). Then hold your breath for as long as you safely can. Next, take a long inhale, and hold your breath for another ten to fifteen seconds. Slowly exhale and repeat two to three times. Not feeling the desired benefits? Then increase the depth and frequency of your breathing, and either repeat the thirty-breath cycle with the hold on the end or switch to deep inhalations through the mouth and exhalations in which you allow the air to come out naturally without pushing.

Wim's approach is much more than simply huffing and puffing; it involves three pillars: gradual cold exposure, breathing techniques, and mind-set. The combination of these principles has been shown to not only influence the autonomic nervous system but reduce inflammation and boost immunity! (Learn more about Wim at Wimhofmethod.com or episode 204 of the Align Podcast.)

Alignment Assignment

For the next thirty days, pay attention to your breath and do your best to make it exclusively come through your nose (unless you're intentionally performing a breath practice that involves mouth breathing). It's OK if you forget sometimes; just gently come back to the nose breathing, and take it easy on yourself.

If you're ever feeling a little congested during your thirty days, try this nose breathing exercise to help clear your nasal passages:

1. Exhale normally through your nose.
2. Pinch your nose with your fingers to hold your breath.
3. While holding your breath, walk at a normal pace until you feel a strong urge to breathe.
4. Breathe in through your nose and calm your breathing as soon as possible.
5. Repeat five times.

CHAPTER 6

Hip Hinging: Give Me Leverage and I'll Move the World

"Intelligent people fix problems. Geniuses prevent them."

—*Albert Einstein*

At a martial arts dojo, the students are clustered around their teacher, a distinguished-looking Japanese man in his sixties. Though they're evidently doing their best to focus on implementing his instructions, they're also growing tired of performing the same movement over and over. Finally, someone speaks up: "Sensei, you've been doing the same technique for an hour. Please show us something different." "You idiot!" Ueshiba replies. "Each and every one was different. When you can perceive the difference, that is when you'll be making progress in aikido."[1] I love this story of the aikido founder scolding his student for missing invaluable attention to detail. It's a beautiful reminder that each moment truly is an opportunity to cultivate your mind, body, and movement if you're running the correct internal programs to do so. This chapter is about movement software and breaking down some key fundamentals that can be used for the rest of your life to keep your body safe, as long as you follow the principles of proper hip and spine mechanics outlined below.

Picking something up from the ground, leaning forward to brush your teeth, chopping vegetables, doing chores, and pushing a chair or some furniture around your house are all excellent opportunities to practice the same principles Ueshiba was advocating for his students by simply bringing more attention to hinging from the hips instead of collapsing forward with the spine. Spinal alignment is critical to ensure your body stays strong and durable, and hinging from the hips carefully and mindfully is a primary step to ensure your body is aligned well. This fundamental movement creates maximum power from your hips, stabilizes your spine, and assists in reorganizing your head, neck, and shoulders back on top of your feet.

If you collapse at any level (e.g., rolled-forward shoulders, head, and spine), the ripple moves up- and downstream from there and becomes a milieu of compensation, which is energetically taxing to maintain. Moshe Feldenkrais, founder of the Feldenkrais Method, referred to this energetic drain via misalignment as "parasitic tension" because these imbalanced patterns are expensive to sustain, pulling from energy stores that could potentially go into performing better in your sport or feeling more energetic with your family.

The few days a week you make it to the gym and heed the basic principles of efficient movement while deadlifting or squatting are a drop in the ocean compared to the remaining 165 hours of the week. If you can begin to implement some of the basic fundamentals of safe and effective movement—such as hinging from the hips—in your daily life, you'll be prepared to move well when it counts. Remember, you're forming your postural patterns constantly, so every moment matters.

ALIGN YOURSELF

When sitting on a typical chair, spend more time on the front of the seat so your torso's weight is on the front edge of your sit bones (ischial tuberosities). If the seat is too low, raise it up so your hips are above the height of your knees by adding cushions or blocks. This will assist in aligning your spine, increasing respiratory efficiency (you'll breathe better), and make you feel more strong and confident. If this becomes tiring, you can prop your mid-back up with cushions to help assist in maintaining the aligned position.

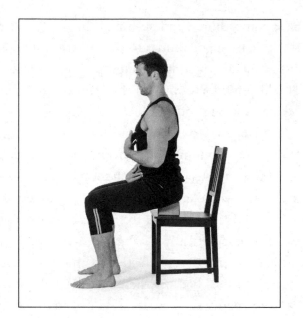

CONTAIN YOURSELF

"Our music is tight but loose."

—Jimmy Page

Our hips are the most robust joint complexes in the human body. They are built to bear hundreds of pounds of pressure. A spine habituated to compressive patterns and lacking support from the hips, not so much. Most of your spinal discs are shaped like little cartilaginous hockey pucks and prefer to not be excessively squashed in a misaligned position while under load. The L5-S1 discs found at the base of your spine are unique in that they're more wedge-shaped, with the wide side of the wedge facing the abdomen toward the front of the body.

Esther Gokhale points out in her book *8 Steps to a Pain-Free Back* that the natural orientation of the spine used to be more of J-shape than the high-amplitude S-curve spine we have become more accustomed to as Westerners.[2] The former is what you commonly see among children before the structural abuse of chair sitting for hours on end begins. In fact, you can even see a difference in the spinal curvature in anatomy charts from the early twentieth century compared to now. Just a hundred years ago, spines were longer, with lower amplitude curves, compared to the present-day "text neck" spines we find commonplace.

An aligned body takes advantage of the natural curve at the base of the spine where the L5 vertebra connects to the sacrum (instead of chronically tucking it under while hunching over in a typical chair) and emphasizes elongation from there to the top of the head. This allows maximal loading with minimal strain by working with the natural shape of your structure instead of against it the way the bucket seat of any car, plane, or bus will do. This is not suggesting that you should allow your whole low back to sway forward into what's referred to as hyperlordosis. The abdomen and low back should stay fully supported in relation to the rest of the torso, like an aligned cylinder, to alleviate any unnecessary stress to the lower back while lifting a weight or even while simply standing and walking. Imagine pressing down on a plastic water bottle that has been bent in the middle and thus collapses at the bend under your downward pressure instead of supporting the weight: Avoid this swaying pattern by lightly tensing your abs with around 20 percent engagement. More strenuous activities such as running or picking up a heavy couch will necessitate greater engagement to support the spine. And you guessed it—less demanding activities like sitting and standing will require lower engagement. This will pull the ribs down toward the pelvis, providing low-back support (like taking the kink out of the water bottle). In fancier terms, you could describe this as maintaining a closed circuit of musculoskeletal connection from your feet to your head in daily movement.

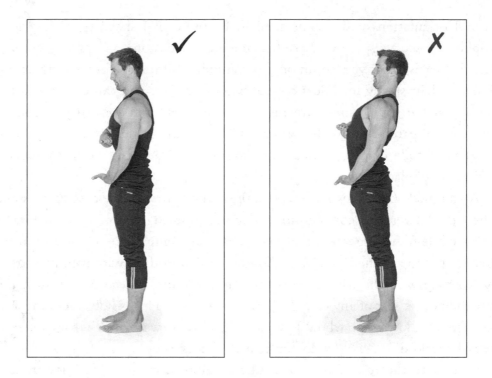

ALIGN YOURSELF

Lie on your back with your knees up so your feet are planted on the ground. Imagine there's a string lightly pulling your low back down to the floor, and press your hands lightly into both sides of your abdomen. Take a deep breath in through your nose and exhale all the air out, making a *sss* or *shh* sound with your mouth. Feel your deep intra-abdominal muscles begin to engage as you get to the end of the exhalation. These deep muscles are somewhat like a corset of support for your spine, and waking them up is foundational for strength, flexibility, and long-term spinal hygiene. Once you master this on the ground, try doing the same thing while standing, and begin integrating this deep abdominal awareness into your daily activities.

BE LIKE SWITZERLAND (STAY NEUTRAL)

"Nothing is worth doing pointlessly."

—*Marcus Aurelius*

A fancy term for the above-mentioned joint balancing act is joint centration, which means the position of greatest contact between the bones to allow for optimal load transfer and maximum muscle contraction during movement. This is essentially referring to a "neutral" position and allows your joints maximum potential for movement in all directions. As the joint transitions out of centration or neutral position, it's like forcing someone's back against a wall. Their options become limited because the ultimatum is injury.

Imagine for a moment the way you'd feel if you were literally being pushed against a wall and the threat of injury was imminent if you made the wrong move. If your joints are misaligned from imbalanced daily movement habits, you're creating this sensation inside your body. Unstable and misaligned joints are inevitably sending signals through the nervous system to become tense as a form of protection because they feel unsafe (i.e., chronically tight neck, shoulders, back, etc.). The chronically held tension isn't because your muscles are just rude—they are doing everything they can to hang on in an unsafe environment (sounds a lot like a partner becoming "clingy" in an unstable relationship; oh, the parallels). I suggest if your joints are sounding alarms of potential danger via imbalance, the mind will be occupied with the noise. Thus, a key to one's mental and emotional health is physical equipoise.

Our tendency to hunch over and jut our heads forward, especially when sitting at a computer, takes the whole body out of balance while putting an immense amount of undue stress on the cervical spine (neck). A regular hip-hinging practice following the principles outlined in this chapter will greatly assist in rebalancing these unsightly patterns. Kenneth Hansraj, a New York back surgeon, calculated this undue neck strain using computer models and found the results to be surprising. The average head weighs ten to twelve pounds, Hansraj wrote. "As the head tilts forward the force seen by the neck surges to 27 pounds at 15 degrees, 40 pounds at 30 degrees, 49 pounds at 45 degrees, and 60 pounds at 60 degrees."[3] If you're feeling like life is "heavy," it may have something to do with the perceived weight of your own body parts being out of alignment. Should your skull be too far in front of the midline, you're effectively lugging around an oversize bobble head all day. No wonder your neck, upper back, and shoulders are always so sore!

ALIGN YOURSELF

Play with this idea of joint stacking by placing a light sandbag (a heavy book will be more challenging but is also an option) on the top of your head and start regularly taking a brisk walk or performing some basic exercises such as lunges or squats while balancing the weight. This will help teach you to maintain length through your spine and neck while hinging the hips to perform the basic exercises.

Aligned Standing (Mountain Pose)

Believe it or not, there is an art and science to just standing around! Let's break down a few "stand-out" pointers to follow.

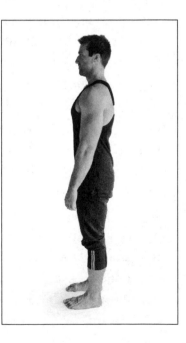

- Maintain a small amount of abdominal engagement to discourage your belly from dumping forward and your lower back from swaying.
- Bring the feet to shoulder width or a slightly narrower position to assist in stacking your bones.
- Imagine there is a string pulling the back of your head up toward the sky, causing your chin to pull slightly backward, allowing your neck to elongate.

■ Observe your breath expanding your ribs out to the sides and filling your belly and low back.

The moment you put excessive stress on any single joint, the whole system suffers the consequences. Not only does it lead to greater potential for injury, but your central nervous system will actually shut down the potential power you could apply during movement out of fear of injury.

Your nervous system is like a protective parent, and the only way it will allow you to wander out to explore is if it has absolute faith you'll be safe. If there is any reason to doubt your safety, you won't be leaving the house, or in this case, picking up heavier objects such as gym weights, grocery bags, furniture, people, pets, or whatever you might be keen to lift.

Dead Lift (Picking Something Up from the Ground)

The fundamentals of this staple weight-lifting movement are consistent in your daily life and are invaluable to master for healthy movement function. Start incorporating these principles into the way you perform chores around the house or move around your office so they become ingrained into your system. A few key points to pay attention to include:

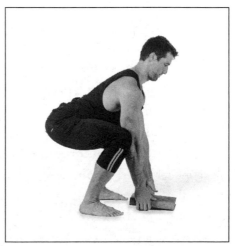

■ Keep your feet facing somewhere between straight ahead to around twelve degrees (think between twelve and one o'clock) of external rotation to allow for optimal hip engagement.

■ Keep the knees over the feet (be sure you can always see your toes) to focus the stress in the hips instead of the knees while lifting.

- Drive the hips backward while maintaining a long, neutral spine (creating a hip hinge).
- Squeeze whatever you happen to be lifting good and tight to recruit as much muscle as you can.
- Start with five to twelve repetitions for three sets with a moderate weight, and be sure to prioritize your form first above all other factors.

MOVEMENT TIP

The dead lift motion to pick something from the ground may not always be the most efficient move; you can basically follow the same fundamental principles mentioned above to lunge down to pick something up as well. The main obvious difference is that you simply step with one leg a couple feet or so back before hinging your hips and bending the knees to descend with a long, neutral spine. Use your breath as a tool while doing so—take a full breath in through the nose on your descent and a full breath out through the nose on your way up. This will help create more tension in your mid-section (yes, sometimes tension is a good thing) to support the spine.

Remember, we are practicing these movement patterns not just for the sake of weight lifting but for lifelong functionality. Notice how these same principles of spine and hip mechanics cross directly over to household activities like hinging forward to brush your teeth, chopping veggies over a low counter, or picking some luggage up from the ground. Begin observing where in your day you can incorporate these simple concepts, and begin feeling your butt come alive, your hips regaining function, and your low back finally healing from those old strains. As you incorporate these

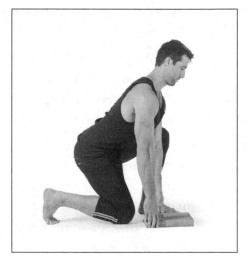

techniques into your daily life, your every moment can become one of repair and strengthening for your whole body!

FIND YOUR FEET

It would be remiss of me to discuss hip and spinal mechanics without mentioning the feet, considering they're the base of the whole structure. As you're squatting, lunging, or just plain hinging over, your foot position is the foundation setting you up for success.

It's of paramount importance to maintain strong contact with all four corners of your feet (I realize feet don't exactly have corners, but you get the point: your big toe, little toe, and both sides of your heel) as you go through these motions. Pay attention to tracking the knees over the second toes, and be sure to sit back enough on your heels so you can see all your toes while keeping them firmly planted on the ground. This will help keep you grounded in your feet while maintaining proper hip engagement. If your knees collapse inward, knee health is compromised, power of the pelvis is reduced, and the output of the hips is mitigated. When you collapse at one point in the body, the compensation ripples throughout the whole.

If the four-points-of-contact position is challenging for you, that's OK; come up with an analogy that works for you to feel your feet well supported by the ground. It's OK to be playful with the visual. If you have certain restrictions, a few simple mobility exercises like rolling a soft ball underfoot or the sitting techniques discussed in Chapter 4, such as sitting on your heels while kneeling (the classic *seiza*) and toe sitting, will help improve the capacity of your feet.

SQUATTING (WHILE HINGING FROM THE HIPS) IS A PART OF YOUR DNA

There has been some debate over the years on whether the full range of a deep squat is in fact healthy for everybody. The answer to this contentious question is as you may expect: It depends on the individual and the technique. There are some basic principles you can follow that will keep you safe for an unloaded deep squat like you'd see as a standard resting position for people in any developing country or a child anywhere around the world. This archetypal resting position may literally be encoded into your genetics. Human fetuses are structurally predisposed to be in a squatting position—you can often see small facet joints develop on the ankles of a fetus while in the womb to permit a child's ankles the range of motion to go into the deep dorsiflexion necessary to a barefoot squat.

The book *Lowly Origins: Where, When, and Why Our Ancestors First Stood Up* by Jonathan Kingdon, a world-renowned zoologist, describes squatting as being an essential part of our evolutionary history. He refers to squatting as a "pre-adaptation" that facilitated a straight spine, allowed us to work and eat from the ground, and was the beginning stage of standing and walking on two feet.[4] The deep squat position acts as a beautiful litmus test for the functional range of motion within your hips, knees, ankles, and pelvic muscles. You can think of this and the other archetypal resting positions we have discussed like computer scanning software for your body to remove unused files and potential viruses while it's at rest.

Nature has designed our bodies in a similar fashion so our resting positions flush out the fluid waste of metabolism, while shaping our joints for optimal functionality when we do decide to get up and move. Kelly Starrett makes a good point with his book *Becoming a Supple Leopard*: A leopard doesn't need to stretch for ten minutes before it is ready to run.[5] This inconvenient quality is strictly human. The reason for this disparity between the human animal compared to other animals is not only that we move less, but our resting positions have mostly been relegated to hunching over as though gravity is that of Jupiter—around two and a half times greater than Earth's, which would make you two and a half times heavier (I felt it was time for a gratuitous astronomy reference; you're welcome). Chronic time spent in this position deharmonizes the orchestra of communication in your muscular system, leaving you feeling heavy and clunky at best.

Tread lightly into the deep squat waters if you fall into the typical chair-sitting Westerner category. Your tissues have taken many years to form into the shape of the chair, seated exercise machines, high-heeled shoes, and chronic standing in place. A few basic principles will keep you safe to re-harness the youthful range of motion you're entitled to.

SQUATTING FUNDAMENTALS

- Keep the knees tracking over the second toe or wider.

- Avoid allowing the knees to drift in front of the toes. You should be able to see your toes during the squat to remove excess stress from the knees.

- A lot of beginners need a tactile cue to know when they've reached sufficient depth, which for the sake of simplicity we'll say is when your thighs are parallel to the ground to start. Then, I recommend you squat as deeply as you can while maintaining the principles discussed in this section.

- Try to pull your hamstrings and butt back to initiate the squat. This will ensure you're engaging your posterior chain (the group of muscles that run along the back of your legs, butt, and back) and not overly relying on your quads.

- Try to maintain tension in your abs throughout the movement to stabilize your torso.

- Do your best to keep your spine upright during the whole movement. I find the goblet squat (see below) to be a helpful practice to cultivate length in the torso.

- Keep the neck long during the whole range of motion, rather than crunching it backward. Imagine a string is pulling the back of your head up toward the ceiling as you squat, creating length all the way down your spine.

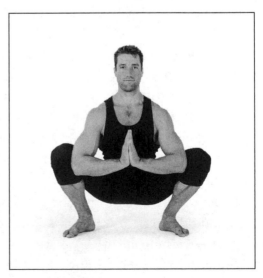

- Try adding more squatting into your day, such as when you need to pick something up from the ground, are waiting at a bus stop, or are getting low to play with an animal or child.

Little by little you can master your resting squat position. If you find this impossible without your heels coming up off the ground, that's fine—just stick with it. You can start by adding a couple of books or a weight plate under your heels to reduce the range of motion necessary for your ankles to squat, and each week drop the height of the books slightly, until eventually you've created enough length to squat with heels on the ground and feet facing straight ahead or just slightly outward.

GLOBAL VS. LOCAL SPINAL CURVES

All this hip hinge and neutral spine talk can create a pathological fear around bending the spine at all. Dr. Roger Sperry, 1981 Nobel Prize winner for brain research, once said, "Ninety percent of the stimulation and nutrition to the brain is generated by the movement of the spine." He would be in agreement that your spine benefits from a vast array of articulations to enrich your health and should not be limited to a single static position, such as permanently being held in a neutral position.

It's OK to bend your spine forward, backward, sideways, or most any direction that feels good; you just need to pay attention to distributing that bend globally through the whole spine, instead of excessively straining locally at a single joint complex, as happens with the classic swayback position or the stress on the cervical spine from forward head posture.

Imagine distributing weight through a fishing pole. You can load the pole up with a decent amount of weight so long as it's loading evenly through the whole rod (global curve). Now imagine bending a fishing pole to a sharp angle in one specific spot (local curve): It will snap with a fraction of the weight added to the former globally curved rod.

Side Note: With the correct breathing techniques to create proper spinal bracing during a lift, it can be safe to lift weight with a globally flexed spine (like a strongman lifting an atlas stone) but for the sake of this book, we are going to stick with hinging the hips with a neutral spine.

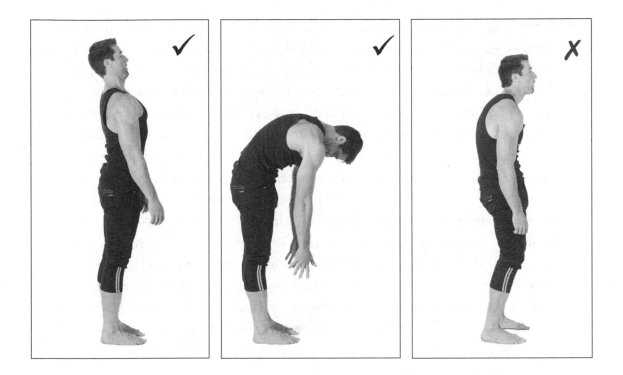

NOT ALL HIPS ARE CREATED EQUAL

While all of our bodies thrive on movement, not all of us are built for the same kind. World-renowned spine expert Dr. Stuart McGill discussed this puzzling concept in detail in a recent Align Podcast episode, and I thought it would be helpful here to shine some light on this common point of confusion. A typical term thrown around among weight-lifting circles is the "Celtic hip" or "Scottish hip," referring to the reduced range of hip motion often found in Celtic populations due to deep hip sockets (acetabulum). A hip joint of this shape is great for walking, standing, and generating rotational power, but its owner may find lifting from the bottom of a deep squat position more challenging to negotiate. These folks will naturally express less hip mobility and are more likely to experience femoral acetabular impingement (FAI), a condition that manifests from too much contact between the ball and socket of the hip joint.

If we jump to the eastern part of Europe, we see a higher concentration of

Olympic lifters emerge and a different hip anatomy to match. Most of the great Olympic weight lifters come from Poland, Bulgaria, and the Ukraine and tend to have a shallow hip socket, leading to greater range of hip motion and greater proficiency at a complex movement like a snatch exercise. The downside of this deep squat superpower is a higher rate of hip dysplasia, a condition where the socket portion doesn't fully cover the ball portion of the femur, leading to joint instability.[6]

Obviously, these are two extreme ends of the spectrum of possible hip anatomy; you likely fall somewhere in between. It's important for you to listen to your own physiology, instead of mimicking an image of someone else on Instagram and jamming yourself into an arbitrary position to your detriment. Remember to always come back to your breath when you are trying a new movement—if you have to hold it and gasp for air, there's a good chance you're in over your head, and it'd be wise to back up to more comfortable terrain. It's an art form getting to know yourself well enough to continually push your boundaries while respecting the limits in place to keep you safe. The road is long—be gradual with the changes you create in your body, and you'll be happier for it in the long run.

ALIGN YOURSELF

There's no use in comparing ourselves as we're too vastly different from one another. Stay focused on what feels best for your own body, free of comparison to the shape of others, and you'll save yourself a lot of energy that you can refocus on your own creativity and doing the best with what you've got anatomically.

Alignment Assignment

For the next thirty days, make hinging from your hips a part of your daily movement: household chores, work, and daily activities. Remember, it's healthy to flex and extend the spine, but try to make it a global flexion and extension through the whole spine instead of a local curve, such as the effect forward head posture has on the neck.

Try this hip hinging sequence to warm yourself up tomorrow morning—or even better, put the book down and start now!

1. Five overhead squats: Reach your arms high overhead while maintaining a long spine and hip hinge for the whole exercise. If you want another option, try to hold the Align Band like a barbell and attempt to pull it apart while turning your arms slightly outward so your thumbs face slightly backward to activate your grip and shoulder girdle muscles during the squats.

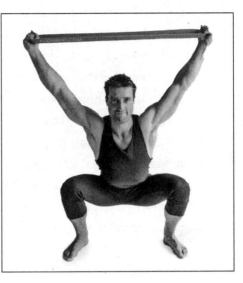

2. Five overhead lunges, following the same principles as the overhead squat.

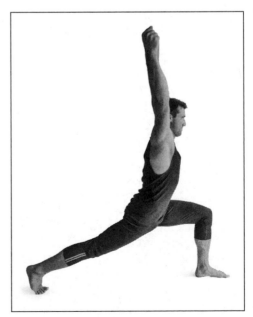

3. Five overhead Good Mornings: Stand tall with your arms reaching overhead (thumbs facing backward) and begin hinging forward at your hips as much as your mobility will allow, while maintaining great form. Your knees can have a slight bend, but your arms should stay straight the whole time (you will feel a strong stretch in your hamstrings). When you get to the low point of each repetition, take a deep breath in and out through your nose before coming back up to stand tall and reaching high again.

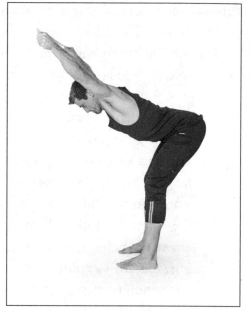

CHAPTER 7

Hanging: The Power of Decompression

"The question of whether we descended from apes, or split from apes, no longer arises, because it hasn't yet happened...We are apes."

—*Richard Leakey in* The Hominid Gang *by Delta Willis*

A key distinction between human beings and other mammals is our capacity to walk upright on two feet. The story becomes extra interesting when you ask, "What the heck were we doing before that?" Our earliest ancestors are believed to have diverged from the common ancestor we share with chimpanzees between 6 and 13 million years ago. A frequently held belief is that climate change shifted our apelike grandparents away from the safety of dwelling within the trees covering much of Africa at the time, out into the savannah.[1]

Other researchers believe becoming bipedal helped our ancestors keep cool in the hot African sun. This would also explain why our ancestors lost the hair from most of their bodies other than the parts that either help send olfactory (smell) signals to potential mates, like the genitals and armpits, or those that protect us from sun, like the top of the head and eyebrows. That's right, your super-cool haircut is likely more of an exaptation (a trait that has been co-opted for a use other than the one for which natural selection built it) evolved for either sun protection or warmth for your noggin.[2]

Regardless of your belief systems around evolution, the human shoulder girdle is built to brachiate (fancy word for "hang"). At a primordial level, human beings are natural hangers, pullers, and curious explorers. Our bodies are designed to navigate through trees (and mountains): A few of these traits include a short spine (particularly the lumbar spine), short fingernails (instead of claws), long curved fingers well suited for grasping, reduced thumbs, long forelimbs, and flexible and freely rotating wrists.[3] Perhaps these traits are remnants from our brachiating ancestors, but more importantly for the purposes of this book, they indicate a biological demand to continue reaching up, hanging, and pulling for optimal health.

When was the last time you hung from something or even stretched your arms over your head? If you're like most people, it's probably been longer than you'd like to admit. If that is the case, you've likely complained of neck, shoulder, or back tension at some point in the last year. Tapping back into your primordial brachiating roots could be the solution!

THERE'S HOPE!

Pioneering orthopedic surgeon Dr. John Kirsch refers to humans as the fifth great ape. The Kirsch Institute conducted a study in 2012 with ninety-two subjects suffering from chronic shoulder pain and found ninety out of ninety-two participants were able to return to comfortable living after implementing a simple daily hanging protocol. Many of these participants avoided surgery and the likelihood of long-term pain with this free and simple intervention.[4] Kirsch is convinced the divergence away from regular hanging is a crucial factor in today's chronic shoulder issues and impingements and claims in his book *Shoulder Pain?* that his simple protocol of regular hanging along with some basic dumbbell exercises will heal 99 percent of shoulder pain.

We're rarely taught this, but even our bones are malleable. There are numerous visible examples of this, from modern baseball pitchers' upper arm bones (humerus) becoming physically altered by the repeated torque of throwing the baseball, to ninth-century European archer skeletons clearly showing greater bony development around the attachments of the dominant archery muscles.[5]

The idea that our bones do in fact change with time and movement is known as Wolff's law, which states that bone grows and remodels in response to the forces that are placed upon it in a healthy person. We find it easy to believe we can move ourselves into a dysfunctional position, but somehow conceive it to be unfathomable to move ourselves back into a balanced posture.

ANATOMICAL BIT...

OK, let me play anatomy professor for just a minute so that I can fully explain why hanging is actually an incredibly important part of realigning your body and returning your strength to its intended level. Hanging creates space within the coracoacromial arch (CA arch), a curved structure in the shoulder that overlies the rotator cuff tendons and includes the coracoacromial ligament. Impingement here is very likely why you may find it painful or challenging to raise your arms straight above your head without swaying your low back forward (resulting in low-back issues—that's right, your low-back thing may actually be a shoulder thing, or vice versa). Hanging stretches the CA arch, expanding the subacromial space, resulting in decompression of these tissues. Our shoulders get stiff and stuck in forward flexion, and regular hanging can not only relieve pain but literally reshape your postural patterns, changing not only the way you look but also the way you think and feel, as explained in the first chapter.

A beautiful description of ape (and human) compared to monkey shoulder anatomy comes from John Gribbin and Jeremy Cherfas in the book *The First Chimpanzee: In Search of Human Origins*:

> By contrast to monkeys, the collar bone of apes (and, of course, man) is longer and helps to keep the shoulder away from the chest. The shoulder is much freer and can move in all sorts of ways; it isn't much of an effort for you to scratch your right ear with your left hand from behind your head, but no monkey could do this...This cluster of adaptations that allows movement by arm-swinging, or brachiation as it is called, is a property only of the apes—gibbons, orangutans, gorillas, chimpanzees and men.[6]

BABY STEPS

For many of you, this might be the first time you've intentionally hung from anything since grade school. If that's the case, it's great news! You'll experience more tangible results from this practice than most other seasoned brachiating people. The key is taking it slowly. You can start simply by simulating hanging from things in front or slightly above you with only as much weight as feels comfortable. Gradually work your way up to hanging from something above your head while keeping your feet on the ground or a bench to support your weight. Eventually you will have worked your way up to a proper hanging position with no additional support beyond your own strength. This is the promised land of maintaining healthy shoulders, neck, spine, grip strength, and tough yet supple hand skin for as long as you occupy your body!

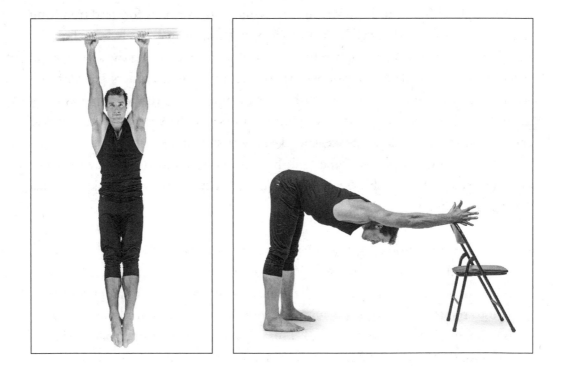

HANGING POINTERS

Get a rock-solid grip: Wrap your fingers as far around the bar as possible and create a strong lock with your thumbs wrapping your index and middle finger. Pretend you are squeezing the pulp out of the bar. Switch between an overhand and underhand grip to explore a full range of motion of the shoulder joint and connective tissue around the forearms. You can vary the width between your hands regularly as well.

Break the bar: As you're hanging with the overhand grip position, alternate between rotating your fists inward and outward as though you're attempting to break the pull-up bar. Put extra emphasis on rotating your fists outward as though you're attempting to point the thumbs behind you. This activates the posterior muscles of the shoulder girdle that need to be strengthened in order to reverse the forward-rolled shoulder pattern.

Strong fingers make strong shoulders: Rotate between emphasizing the pressure on each finger, as all the digits will activate different muscles through your arms and shoulders. Also, alternate between squeezing the bar as tightly as possible with all your fingers and coming back into a more relaxed grip; hanging can be very dynamic, as you may be finding out!

Engage the belly (hollow position): The tendency for many people is to allow the abdomen to sway forward, borrowing motion from the lower back that you couldn't find in the shoulders. Avoid this by pointing the toes, slightly raising your feet in front of you and drawing your low ribs to your hips as though knitting up your abdomen with a corset. You could also picture your pelvis as a wineglass and you pouring the wine back behind you (don't spill it out the front of the cup and ruin your nice carpet!).

YOU'RE SO CALLUS

Your skin is an essential part of your kinetic chain of movement, and you're only as strong as your weakest link. For many people, the weak links are skin and grip strength (or lack thereof). I can't help but feel a little bit more badass every time I put on a pair of motorcycle gloves, as though some biker gang alter ego emerges momentarily. This sensation is likely similar to how folks in the gym feel wearing gloves to protect their hands from the abrasion of bars, kettlebells, and dumbbells. What they may not realize is they're in fact wearing a crutch that in the long run is impeding their full-body (including skin) strength and adaptation to the movements in a natural setting. If you've adapted your muscles to movements your skin strength is not adequately robust enough to support, you are not truly adapted for the movement you're practicing in the gym.

This could be equated to taking a basic town car with cheap, skinny tires and replacing the engine with that of a Formula One race car. When you take it to the track, it'll be all kinds of loud but won't effectively distribute the engine's power to the road, leaving the car spinning its cheap tires, losing traction until eventually they blow out. The analog to this tire blowout in the human body is the formation of a blister, which comes as a product of new friction where the body did not have adequate time to toughen the skin through the process of callusing.

The skin of your palms and feet, known as glabrous (smooth and hairless), ridged skin, and/or thick skin, is built for friction. The rough, callused skin that shows up after activities like hanging is thought by many to be dead skin, but it's quite the opposite. It has increased circulation, and the tissue has formed a cross-link pattern, making it more durable to protect against future damage. Spending time working with your hands essentially makes your hands smarter, stronger, and more dependable.[7]

GET A GRIP

Grip strength doesn't really matter for anything other than occasionally crushing a can as a bar trick, right? It turns out a lack of grip strength is associated with heart attacks, stroke, and cardiovascular disease—three of the top five biggest killers in the United States. As a part of the international Prospective Urban and Rural Epidemiological (PURE) study, researchers calculated grip strength using a dynamometer for almost 140,000 people from 17 different countries and observed their health for an average of four years after.[8]

Here's where it gets creepy: They found each eleven-pound decrease in grip strength to be associated with 17 percent higher risk of dying from heart disease, 9 percent higher risk of stroke, 7 percent higher risk of heart attack, and a 16 percent higher risk of dying from any cause. Grip strength was an even better predictor of death or cardiovascular disease than blood pressure! It turns out, one of the key factors to being harder to kill is maintaining a grip on life.[9]

Statistics like this can become perverted quickly, with people attempting to isolate their grip strength in prevention of cardiovascular disease. Grip strength is actually better developed holistically by doing manual work that involves grabbing, pulling, climbing, or hanging. That's right, it's better to actually do activities involving grip strength than to try to hack your heart health by isolating your can-crushing muscles. You could join a climbing gym, start a garden, do yard work more regularly, or just start hanging on random branches as you're out for a walk!

ALIGN YOURSELF

The farmer's carry exercise is one of the more valuable "functional" movements to strengthen your grip strength in a natural way. It's very simple: Grab a couple heavy weights (this could include paint cans, kettlebells, dumbbells, or anything you can hold on to) and take a walk for thirty seconds or so. Pay attention to gripping evenly through all your fingers and imagine you're squeezing the pulp out of the handles as you walk. Follow the same principles described in the Aligned Standing (mountain pose) exercise from Chapter 6. Stay calm and breathe through the nose. Your heart will thank you in a few years!

SPINAL DECOMPRESSION

Low-back pain caused by musculoskeletal conditions costs Americans more than $100 billion each year, and more than 80 percent will experience it at some point in their lives.[10] Our modern lives are inherently compressive to the discs of our spines due to an overabundance of sitting in dysfunctional positions, sedentary lifestyles that inhibit fluid from freely circulating throughout our tissues, and, I would suggest, a lack of decompression time spent hanging. Continually sitting with pelvis tucked under like a sad puppy puts continual tension on the hockey puck–shaped discs between your vertebrae. Not to mention this position chronically shortens the muscle in the front of the hip, forming you into a ticking time bomb for low-back problems, and plopping you into the 80 percent or $100 billion category mentioned above. This painful fate is absolutely avoidable, and a daily hanging practice is a key part of the remedy.

In Pavel Tsatsouline's powerful book *Relax into Stretch*, he recommends hanging from a pull-up bar with weight around your waist to assist with decompressing the spine.[11] This is a nice technique because it adds an extra subtle pull through the spine, thus bringing new healthy fluid to tissues in and around the vertebral discs while flushing out the old stuff. Our spines are bearing some serious weight throughout the day, especially when you start asymmetrically loading them up with things like purses, briefcases, backpacks, and things of the sort. Multiply the awkward loads we carry by the chronic hunching over from chair sitting, cell phone staring, and couch reclining, and you have a spine crying out to be decompressed with a good hang.

DECOMPRESSION TIPS

Contract-relax: As you are hanging, alternate between squeezing your grip super tight for five seconds and then relaxing as much you can while holding on to the bar. Do the same with your shoulder girdle by pulling your shoulders down and lifting your body up, while keeping your arms straight. This motion is technically called depression and retraction of the scapula. Think of pulling your scapulae (shoulder blades) down and toward the spine, contracting to about 80 percent for five seconds, and then relaxing back into a passive hang for ten seconds. Repeat this for as many reps as you can maintain good form.

Breathe: A key to getting the most out of your hang time, like everything else, goes back to your quality of breath. Gray Cook, founder of the Functional Movement Screen (FMS), pretty much sums it up by saying, "If you can't control your breath, you can't control your movement."[12] Hanging is no different, so pay attention to moving your breath into the various parts of your torso, neck, shoulders, and hips. Each breath in assists in expanding your various parts, and the breath out is a release of tension in those areas.

Key Points

- The anatomy of the human shoulder girdle is built to brachiate (hang)—it has very likely been a primary component of human evolution.
- You can literally change the structure of the shoulder girdle to restore function and reduce or eliminate pain with a simple daily hanging protocol.
- If free-hanging is too much, you can replicate the effects of hanging by reaching your arms over your head and stretching them on the end of a chair.
- One of the most effective ways to decompress your spine is to regularly get some hang time in each day.

Alignment Assignment

You didn't think I'd just leave you hanging (dad joke) without providing some actionable homework to cultivate those brachiating shoulders of yours, did you?

For the next ten days (at least), find a way to hang for a total of ninety seconds to three minutes (depending on your fitness level) each day. This means you could hang for thirty seconds three to six times or fifteen seconds six to twelve times, or whatever works best for you. Find equipment at your gym, monkey bars at a playground, a strong tree branch, or another sturdy place to get your hang time in. I recommend buying a pull-up bar to place in a doorway you walk through regularly in your home and gifting yourself a brief shoulder-opening, spine-decompressing hang each time you walk through. This will become something you look forward to. These simple and consistent habits over extended periods of time are truly age-defying. Enjoy!

CHAPTER 8

Walking: Circulating Your Mind and Body

"In every walk with nature one receives far more than he seeks."

—*John Muir*

In his bestselling book *Blue Zones*, Dan Buettner identifies commonalities between the daily rituals, habits, and lifestyles of the people around the world who live the longest and with the greatest vitality. One thing they all share is walking outside. In his research for the *National Geographic* series that eventually formed the basis for his book, Buettner found that Sardinian shepherds walk five miles a day up and down steep hillsides, the most of any of the Blue Zones inhabitants.[1]

The links between frequent walking, longevity, and quality of life aren't limited to Buettner's project. Recent findings from the American Cancer Society's widespread study of 140,000 people showed that those who walk at least six hours per week have a significantly lower risk of developing respiratory disease, cancer, and cardiovascular complaints. And just two hours of walking per week moved the needle on all three diseases in a positive direction.[2] Clearly, one of the easiest ways to live longer and more healthfully is to simply take a daily stroll (ideally outside in nature if you have access).

Craig Stanford states in his enlightening book *Upright* that the current structure of the human body would not exist had our ancient ancestors not literally stood up for themselves. "The modern architecture of the spine, pelvis, feet, and hands, and even nervous and circulatory systems, follows directly from the conversion from quadrupedalism to bipedalism," Stanford asserts.[3]

He goes on to identify three major benefits of becoming bipeds: the ability to travel long distances to search for food, more successful hunting of prey, and the capacity to carry children, weapons, and tools. These factors formed the bedrock for a fundamental social shift, whereby our forebears not only hunted and foraged far and wide, but also came into contact with other tribes, discovered new lands, and conquered both.[4]

OK, history lesson over. We're done recapping millennia of human development; what's the relevance of all this for us today? Simply put, along with breathing, walking is one of the most fundamentally human things we can do and deserves our attention, with a caveat: All walking (and breathing) is not created equal.

THE ART AND SCIENCE OF WALKING

All this "walk more" stuff sounds great and all, but what if you're a person who tends to get knee or hip pain after walking for any extended period of time, as though there's a friction fire happening between your joints? Or perhaps you get tired quickly and feel as though your legs are filled with lead while you watch kids elastically bounce by. What is this elastic quality of movement?

These springy folks are all accessing their built-in elastic recoil qualities during movement. Let's say you set out for a walk or run. The very first step you take going from zero to one uses the most energy because of the need to overcome inertia and transition from being stationary to in motion (sounds a lot like creating momentum in starting a new healthy habit). Once you're on the move, notice what your arms and hips do. As you get into the rhythm, your opposite arm and hip pull away from each other on each step (in fancy speak, this is called contralateral motion). Imagine you had a rubber band connected from each of your shoulders to the opposite ankle that wrapped down both the front and back of your body. Each step you take lengthens those bands to spring you back in the other direction. After you've started the process of loading your internal stretchy bands (primarily tendons, but they also include muscles, ligaments, and connective tissues), they sling you back into the next step in large part via the stored energy from the previous step.[5] Pretty clever design, right?

Think of your musculoskeletal system like strings of a guitar: Each step you take is a strumming of the chords. If the chords are aligned and tuned, the body plays with harmony. If any single string is too tight, loose, long, or short, the song you play in the world will sound a little bit *off*. The cacophony of imbalance translates biologically to a whole host of compensatory patterns—joint pain, higher stress levels, discomfort in your own body, trouble with self-expression, increased likelihood of injury, etc.

If your strings are slightly out of sync for walking with optimal efficiency, that's OK, there's hope! Start using these fundamental self-care practices to bring them back into balance and you'll begin to feel more connection. Feel free to visit www.TheAlignBook.com for detailed video instructions on these techniques and more!

SELF-CARE FOR BETTER WALKING

Ankle Mobilization (with Band)

Your ankle mobility is key to a successful gait pattern, hip mobility, and spinal health. If there is restriction in the ankle, it will block the hip from extension (moving backward while walking), causing problems through the whole body. Attach the Align Band to a door (or whatever you have handy) as low to the ground as you can and wrap the band around the front of your ankle. Walk yourself away from the door to create tension in the band, and step away with your opposite foot, putting you

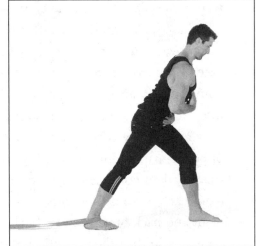

in a traditional runner's stretch while using the band to decompress the ankle joint. Keep the back heel on the ground the whole time to lengthen the posterior muscles of your leg and foot. Hold for approximately ninety seconds on each ankle, and feel free to use the techniques mentioned in Chapter 3 such as Contract-Relax.

Lunge (with Band)

Raise the door anchor of the Align Band to just above hip height and wrap the band around the hip on the forward-stepping leg. Step away from the door to create tension in the band and step your front foot about three or four feet away from the back or until you feel a stretching sensation in the back hip. Follow the same lunging principles mentioned in Chapter 6. Once you are in the lunge, you can raise your arms overhead and rotate your torso to the opposite side of the back leg to create more of a stretch through the hip and torso (optional to pass the band around the back stepping leg as well for greater focus on deeper hip extension). Hold for approximately thirty seconds and switch legs, remembering to breathe.

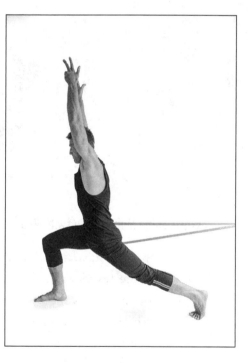

Banded Quad Stretch

Bring yourself into lunge position with your feet about two or three feet apart and drop your back knee down onto a pillow or cushion. Wrap the Align Band around the back foot and use it pull your knee into flexion, lengthening the front of the hip and quadriceps muscles. Lightly pull upward on the band to create a deeper stretch, and remember to breathe. Hold this position for about ninety seconds and alternate, using the Contract-Relax technique mentioned in Chapter 3.

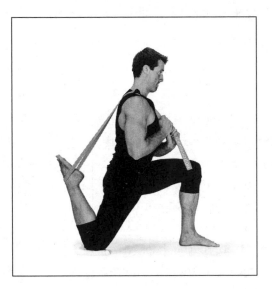

Thoracic Spine Mobilization (with Band)

This is one of my favorite spine mobility techniques (shown opposite). Face the door and place the door anchor at heart level. Pass the band around your spine at that same height. Walk yourself backward until you feel moderate tension in the band creating a pull forward on your thoracic spine. Raise your arms overhead with your thumbs facing backward and feel your breath pushing outward against the tension of the band. Squat as deeply as is comfortable while maintaining a long, neutral spine, and begin slowly twisting your torso to the left and right. Hold on each side for about the length of a full breath. Alternate sides five times or as much as feels good for you!

Now that we've explored the physical facets of walking, we're about ready to move on to the cognitive component. Taking a walk isn't just good for your body, but can also be enriching for your mind.

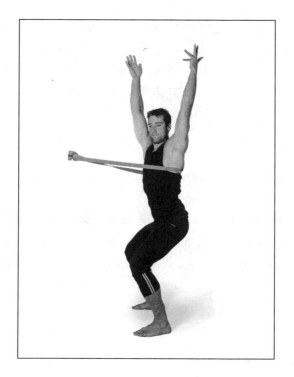

I'M WALKING, YES INDEED, AND I'M TALKING

So sang blues legend Fats Domino, and his words still ring true over half a century later. Fast-forward fifty years and switch from the swamps of the Louisiana bayou to the brush of Silicon Valley, and we find Steve Jobs in his trademark black turtleneck strolling across Apple's California campus, deep in conversation with the company's design guru Jony Ive. What could they be discussing? Perhaps the design of the click-wheel iPod, iPhone, iPad, or iSomething that was soon to take over our lives.

Jobs realized early on in his second stint at Apple that holding meetings in his office or a conference room made him feel like a caged lion. So he started making just about every exchange with his colleagues and minions a walking one. Though, sadly, he didn't live to see it, Jobs worked closely with the architects who designed the new Apple headquarters to create the infinite, walking-friendly loop at the heart of the $5 billion campus. And perhaps just as meaningfully, Jobs was adamant that his legacy should be found not only in gloriously simple electronic devices, but also in the 9,000 drought-tolerant trees (he consulted with an arborist, as one does), myriad plants, a walled garden, and a meadow—all in place before any employees moved into their new work digs.[6]

ALIGN YOURSELF

Seize every opportunity to bust out of those PowerPoint-afflicted meeting rooms and take your back-and-forth with your coworkers outside. Second, be intentional about where you're walking, listen actively, and enjoy natural pauses when your conversation ebbs, rather than trying to fill every second with talking.

A WALK TO REMEMBER

An important and unsung benefit of walking that typically strides under the radar is its ability to improve memory consolidation and recollection. If you've ever taken a walk to clear your head or have had a "Eureka!" moment when out taking a stroll, you'll know what I'm referring to. A study published in the *American Journal of Health Promotion* concluded that those subjects who walked for fifteen minutes at a moderate pace before a learning exercise encoded the lesson more effectively than the ones who didn't, as was shown by their greater recall when tested later.[7]

The connection between taking a walk and enhancing memory also extends to preventing or even reversing age-related mental decline. A *Proceedings of the National Academy of Sciences* paper compared three groups of people ages fifty-five to eighty who had previously lived sedentary lifestyles. One group walked for forty minutes three times a week, the second did yoga, and the third performed band-based resistance training exercises. When studying scans of all three groups, the scientists discovered that the walking group had undergone a positive neurological change: Their hippocampuses had grown by an average of 2 percent.[8]

While a small percentage, this actually has big implications, as the hippocampus is responsible for memory formation and recall. (Fun fact: The word "hippocampus" is derived from the Greek *hippokampus*: *hippos*, meaning "horse," and *kampos*, meaning "sea monster," because the structure resembles a seahorse.)[9] The researchers stated that the six months of thrice-weekly walks had reversed age-related memory loss by one to two years.[10] Another study at the University of British Columbia found similar results when the 120 minutes of brisk weekly walking was divided into just two sessions.[11]

ALIGN YOURSELF

If you've got a big test or presentation coming up, or anything for which you'd like your mind especially sharp, take a brief, mid-paced stroll beforehand. Combine this with walking at a rapid clip for at least two hours total each week. While you're at it, toss some dance moves and music in there for bonus brain juice.

SEEKING SPIRITUAL CONNECTION

"No one saves us but ourselves. No one can and no one may. We ourselves must walk the path."

—*Buddha*

For millennia, people across all faith traditions—including those with a faith in science—have benefited from starting each day with a thoughtful walk. I felt the profound impact of walking with intention while staying at a Vipassana Meditation Center near Joshua Tree, California, with nothing to do between sessions sitting on a cushion other than taking a walk around the desert path they had formed for meditators. I felt a profound sense of connection with the unspoiled landscape, which, despite its dryness, has a haunting beauty that's all its own. There is magic in every step, no matter the environment; we just tend to miss it when we live all the way up in our heads so far from the ground.

In his bestselling book *The Rise of Superman*, Steven Kotler explores the way that extreme athletes, most of whom are performing their feats in the outdoors, are able to readily access flow regularly. Yet it's not just the Tony Hawks, Laird Hamiltons, and Paige Almses of the world who can find flow in nature—it's accessible to the rest of us mere mortals, too. Why? Because the great outdoors contains by its very nature (pun intended) three of the main flow state triggers: novelty, complexity, and variability. And you don't have to be going over a waterfall, BASE jumping off the side of a mountain, or towing into a seventy-foot wave to access such triggers. In fact, the simple act of taking a walk by yourself, going on a bike ride with a friend, or hiking with your family can put you in a state of deep and satisfying embodiment in which time flies and you're at your most creative.

Such outside immersion also has lasting positive effects once you head back indoors. A study by Dr. Chuck Hillman at the University of Illinois used fMRI imaging to compare the brains of two groups. One group did twenty minutes of seated meditation, while the other took a twenty-minute walk. While the scans of the post-meditation brains showed an uptick in activity in several regions, the post-perambulation brains were lit up like a July Fourth fireworks display.[12] It's no wonder, then, that many creative people, from Charles Dickens to Beethoven to Aristotle, swore by taking a daily walk. It literally ignited their minds, and it can do the same to stoke your creativity, too.

ALIGN YOURSELF

If getting into a flow state is your goal, release the idea of multitasking. Try to find a time in your day that comes either right before you're typically at your most productive so you can amplify this output, or use mindful walks to give you a boost during lulls. If you're an early bird, see if you can carve out space for a silent, solitary walk some mornings. More of a night owl, or somewhere in between? Find a time in the afternoon where you can take a break in your day to walk. Resist the temptation to pull out your phone—there's nothing calming or sacred about cruising your (anti)social media feeds, and you'll be amazed at what you start to hear when you're not using earbuds or headphones to create your own isolation chamber.

GET LOST!

I mean that with the utmost respect. Every once in a while, make time in your life for a good old-fashioned wander. You might want to leave the GPS/smartphone/fitness tracker at home (or at least in your pocket) and try to find your own way. While there is benefit to using a map and compass (it's a skill, after all), even those hearty wilderness and urban explorers who've been doing it awhile eventually progress to a more independent version, whereby they just head out and see where they end up.[13]

"But why would I try to get lost?" I hear you ask. Well, you wouldn't, not exactly. Rather, you'd just start to reclaim some of that inbuilt directional sense that's hardwired into us as a survival instinct, rather than always abdicating your route planning to Siri. I'm not making this up. A McGill University experiment found that people who navigate spatially had more activity in the hippocampus than those who relied on a stimulus-response method (like using their smartphone's navigation tool).[14]

ALIGN YOURSELF

If you're planning to go somewhere and are likely to revisit soon, try to memorize the route or use landmarks and street signs to figure out how to get there and back. You can always bring your phone or fire up in-car GPS if things go awry and your poor, atrophied hippocampus fails to see you right. But going back to a paper map occasionally might be a good, brain-stimulating halfway house between finding your own way and letting your nav do all the work for you. This is because, said McGill University's Veronique Bohbot, making sense of that old road atlas "is difficult, it's complicated, it's demanding."[15] All the better for your brain.

TAKING THE ROAD LESS FLATTENED

"I think that I cannot preserve my health and spirits, unless I spend four hours a day at least—and it is commonly more than that—sauntering through the woods and over the hills and fields, absolutely free from all worldly engagements."

—*Henry David Thoreau*

From city sidewalks to office corridors to those moving walkways in airports (I actually quite enjoy those things), we rarely encounter any kind of gradient or texture when we walk. Plus, these flat surfaces are also hard, which is one of the reasons road runners insist on putting an inch or two of cushioning foam between their feet and the pavement they pound, effectively muting one of the most potent input channels in the human body.

So what's the big deal? Well, at the risk of being repetitive, the human foot was not designed to be locked into super-cushioned shoes with chunky heels, arch supports, "motion control" features, and all the other gimmicks companies have told us are essential. We also weren't built to stick to featureless paths that don't offer any kind of stability challenge to our thirty-three joints. Because we've coddled our feet too much, they've become weak and immobile, leading to millions spent each year in podiatry offices, and contributing to the billions spent annually on low-back pain.

The cure? Seek out inclines and declines that are challenging to the feet and ankles, go diagonally or in a zigzag pattern across hills rather than straight up and down them, and head off-road whenever possible. Walk barefoot on the beach, in grass, and on other soft natural surfaces, which will have the dual benefit of strengthening and mobilizing your feet. If you don't have access to a safe public area for walking sans shoes, use your backyard if you have one. Shed your socks when you're walking around the house. When you have to wear shoes, go for a pair with a thin, flexible midsole with no more than four millimeters heel-to-toe drop, as these will be best for your feet. Forgo flip-flops, though: Keeping them on your feet requires you to overengage your toes, which will only make you tighter and less mobile (sandals with heel straps are fine). Leonardo Da Vinci wrote, "The human foot is a masterpiece of engineering and a work of art." While my gnarly toes don't deserve a display in the Tate Modern, binding them up in clunky shoes and lurching around on concrete is not what they were made for. It's time to set your feet free!

ALIGN YOURSELF

Natural movement expert Katy Bowman recommends seeking out walking routes that require you to leave well-beaten paths and crunch through leaves, ford streams, and clamber over fences. She also suggests shedding your shoes whenever possible so you get real-time feedback from your feet, which have more nerves per square inch than any other body part.[16] If you are going to wear shoes, choose a brand like Joe Nimble, Vivo-Barefoot, or Lems, which make flexible options with minimal heel-to-toe drop and toe boxes wide enough to give your feet some breathing room—bunions, hammer toes, and all.

SENSORY DEPRIVATION

A point rarely spoken of in relation to the endemic issue of low-back pain and injury is the sudden sensory deprivation of our feet in recent history. Your feet are massively represented on the sensory cerebral cortex, along with the eyes, ears, nose, hands, nipples, and genitals. Your feet—along with these other super-sensitive body parts—happen to stem embryologically from a common location referred to as the Wolffian ridge. When you go barefoot or wear minimal shoes with thin soles, your feet receive micro-feedback from the ground about the density, curvature, gradient, and other elements of the surface you're interacting with underfoot. This allows you to make tiny adjustments to your balance and posture that are appropriate for your environment.

However, in the past few hundred years we've taken to putting layers of foam and rubber under our feet, cutting them off from the connection to the ground and the subtle recalibrations a bare foot would make moment to moment. As a result, our feet are weaker, less mobile, and less sensitive than they have been at any point in human history. Air soles, motion-control plates, and arch supports might seem cool in shoe ads, but they're silencing the rich sensory feedback that the 7,000 nerve endings in each foot should be providing to the brain and nervous system every time we make contact with the ground. Depriving your feet of the natural stimuli that they have received for millennia may also very well be directly associated to low-back issues experienced by the majority of Westerners. Phillip Beach wrote extensively about these connections in his book *Muscles and Meridians* and said this about the back-foot connection:

> The most vulnerable spinal segments are found at the junctional area of the lumbar spine and the sacrum (L4/L5 and S1), which send their sensory spinal nerves down to the soles of the feet, i.e., the most vulnerable segments are driven by the most information. This is important. The small muscles of the low back are thus segmentally related to the soles of the feet. Information drives all systems, so here we have a sensory platform devoted to the most vulnerable region of the low back. Shoes, from this perspective, are sensory deprivation chambers that cut down the raw information we need to stand and walk in our precarious upright manner."[17]

ALIGN YOURSELF

Grab a few good size rocks to have around your yard to walk and balance on each day. Be barefoot at home—inside and outside—whenever you can. Take advantage of nature when you have the opportunity and be quicker to pop your shoes off when you walk past a grassy patch. Embrace being the weirdo balancing on the root of a tree barefoot. You can tell people you're rehabbing the years of desk-sitting trauma you experienced in grade school.

CIRCULATION STATION

You may have heard the catchy sound bite, "Sitting is the new smoking," credited to Dr. James Levine in the book *Get Up!* While this might initially seem a bit alarmist, it's not actually inaccurate, but neither does it tell the whole story. Our largely seated lifestyles have perpetuated an obesity epidemic, sent rates of diabetes and cardiovascular disease soaring, and robbed us of our vitality, this is true. As discussed in Chapter 4, a gaping hole in this conversation is *the way in which you sit*—it's not as much about the quantity as it is the quality and the micro-movements in between. Instead of being glued to chairs, the simple acts of spending more time eating, working, and hanging out on the ground, along with walk breaks in between, are a primary solution to the symptoms associated with the so-called sitting epidemic (see Chapter 4 for the specifics on how and why).

A core dilemma with excessive chair sitting is that it puts your lymphatic system, which is meant to pump out waste products, into sleep mode; unlike the cardiovascular system, which pumps automatically via the heart, the lymphatic system requires movement. University of Utah researchers recently sought to find a minimum effective dose for during-the-day movement. They discovered that people who walked as few as two minutes every hour reduced their risk of premature death by a third.[18]

This isn't a shocker, as the lymphatic and immune systems are best mates, like Batman and Robin, for keeping you healthy. The Columbia University Medical Center noted that people who replaced thirty-five minutes of sitting with physical activity of any kind or intensity cut their mortality risk by up to 35 percent.[19] All this talk of death getting you down? Well, it shouldn't: The good news from both these studies is that all you need to do to stay alive longer is to stand up and get moving more often with the simplest of all exercises: walk.

While it's great to take an extended walk each day, try to fit in micro-movement, too. Can't remember to get up from your desk or couch and walk around, do some jumping jacks, or get outside? Set a timer! Then download an app like Move, Stand Up!, or Stretchy to remind you, or use your fitness tracker for the same purpose.

Alignment Assignment

For the next thirty days, intentionally make more opportunities to go for walks and pay attention to the way it feels as you do so! Instead of meeting people for coffee, meet for a walk (feel free to grab a cup of coffee or tea and bring it along).

Try this mobility technique before you go to bed tonight as well. I refer to it as the Venus Fly Trap: Simply place the individual fingers of your right hand in between each toe on the left foot (the pattern of finger, toe, finger, etc., clasped together looks a bit like a Venus fly trap) and begin using your hand to stretch open the toes in all directions for about two minutes. Then switch to do the same with the left hand working with your right foot.

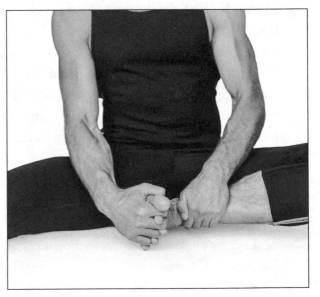

PART III

YOUR ENVIRONMENT FORMS YOUR MIND AND BODY

CHAPTER 9

Clothing—If the Shoe Fits

"Beauty is not in the face; beauty is a light in the heart."

—*Kahlil Gibran*

Have you ever thought about the potential downstream effects of "binding" your hips and knees with tight pants, limiting your full range of motion in a squat, for example? Squatting is not just a gym-based exercise, but a fundamental position essential to the health of your daily physiology. Think of it more like drinking water than an "exercise."

What would happen if you drank all your water for the week on Monday morning over at Gold's Gym in a hard forty-five-minute hydration session? It wouldn't look pretty is the answer, and it's a similar story with the biological staple we call squatting. It's best to wear pants or shorts that allow you to squat regularly and easily with full range of motion all the time. In fact, there was a time not too long ago that these two activities would often happen in tandem; e.g., squatting by a river or spring to gather water, and then drinking it (see just about any *National Geographic* documentary on indigenous peoples).

Squatting, lunging, and walking are some of the major players in moving fluids through your body. The majority of your organs do not have onboard muscles to function, but instead are dependent on pressure regulation from your movement to operate and keep you healthy. Squatting changes the pressure in your abdomen and circulates fluids that otherwise would be stagnant. This chain of pressure-based events takes place because your body is a closed hydraulic system.

What the heck does all that mean? Move one part of the body, and the effect ripples through the whole system like a tube of toothpaste when you squeeze the end. We are essentially an elaborate collection of pumps moving fluid from one compartment to the next. Our overall health is related to the level in which we move our internal fluids. The movement of our internal fluids is dependent on our ability to regularly move through a full range of motion (ROM), and our ROM is limited by the pants we wear!

TAKE THE SQUAT TEST

The squat test involves nothing more than taking your legs through a healthy range of motion to be sure your pants don't impede you from becoming a stronger, more flexible version of yourself.

From this point forward, before purchasing a new skirt, pair of pants, or shorts, see if you can squat in them. If you are limited in your ability to go through your full leg ROM with the pants you own, choose a different pair. If you wear clothes you can move in, you will move better and more!

FOOTWEAR (AND WHY IT MATTERS)

Your feet are the foundation for your body, and if any part of the feet is compromised, the whole system compensates, leading to imbalance and tension. In the practice of Rolfing Structural Integration, a form of manual therapy that systematically balances the body from foot to head, practitioners like me begin to "reorganize" the feet very early on when working with new clients. Why is this?

Let's start by taking a brief anatomical glance at the foot. A quarter of the bones in the whole body are in the feet alone; that's 26 bones, 33 joints, 117 ligaments, and 19 muscles per foot. With this knowledge, it seems fairly apparent that we've naturally evolved to have a wide variety of lower limb movement. For any folks who are into math, those thirty-three foot joints allow us 8.6×10^{36} different foot positions, translating to a zillion options of motion. It almost feels criminal to shut down that beautiful potential by wearing excessively tight, rigid, or high heel–supported footwear. Our feet, like the rest of our body, are continually adapting to the environment we drop them in.

If we cram ourselves into a rigid environment, like when we consistently wear poor-fitting or restrictive shoes, our growth potential is stunted, and compensatory patterns echo throughout the body as a whole. Hopefully this provides new meaning the next time your local crystal-slinging "spiritual" person suggests, "It's all connected." If there's one clothing article we should be examining diligently for structural health and longevity, shoes likely take the cake. Let's take a look at a few relevant factors to observe in purchasing a shoe that supports ease, flexibility, strength, and comfort for your hounds. They work hard for you and deserve the best!

WIDE TOE BOX

Have you ever had the sensation of going on a vacation someplace warm and noticed your feet literally grow in size? Excluding the chance you were recently stung by a jellyfish, this is likely because your feet literally expand to their natural dimension when spending time walking barefoot or in open shoes on varied surfaces, like the beach, rocks, or grass. If the muscles of the feet are able to relax and find their own natural support, you start that same trend in the rest of the body. Try it now. Stand up and scrunch your feet against the ground. You will notice a contraction traveling up your legs, all way up to the back of your neck. Temporary contraction is a great thing. However, chronic contraction is a serious liability. If you maintain this scrunch for an extended period of time, you will notice the positive sensation of the contraction will fairly quickly turn into one of exhaustion and excess tension.

Your shoes should permit you to spread open your toes as wide as you can. Anything shy of full foot range of motion is similar to wearing a foot cast after an injury—with repeated use, they become more like foot coffins. After wearing the foot cast, you would need to go through months of rehabilitation to recover healthy range of motion and muscular support. An eerily high percentage of modern footwear has been "binding" our feet—to a lesser degree than during China's Song Dynasty, but binding nonetheless. It's both sad and fascinating to think that throughout history, beauty has somehow become conflated with pain.

ROLL IT UP

The Tarahumara tribe from Copper Canyon in northern Mexico, brought into the popular consciousness by Christopher McDougall's book *Born to Run*, are some of the world's most elite runners, and like most running tribes across the globe, they choose the simplest of foot protection. They find anything more supportive than sandals made from a thin piece of rubber tire impedes their ability to access their own natural movement mechanics. And these guys aren't just going for a jog around the block—they routinely run dozens of miles across the Mexican desert.

When looking for a favorable shoe, the roll-up test is a good starting point. It should be fairly easy to roll the toe of the shoe up to touch the back. If not, you are likely outsourcing your own foot muscles and growing dependent on the support structure of the shoe, leading to muscular atrophy and a whole host of ankle, knee, hip, and back problems upstream. This is not a huge problem for a short time (like heels), but prolonged use of those shoes will weaken your feet, leading to a dependency on excessively supportive footwear.

DITCH THE HEELS (USUALLY)

It turns out ankle range of motion is not just a foot thing but a brain thing, too! Before you get your feathers ruffled, hear me out. Walking activates mechanoreceptors in the lower extremities, stimulating cerebello-thalamo-cortical loops in the brain (I'm not making that term up, I promise). The reduced cortical activity changes dopaminergic function, which is associated with the way you think and feel.[1] Wait, what? Yeah, my brain hurts from just typing that; essentially what it's saying is that research shows you need to move your ankles for your brain to function optimally and your mental health to stay in check.

If you're still thinking that a great new pair of shoes makes you happy enough to counteract the lack of ankle movement, how about we focus on something that about 80 percent of Americans will experience in their lifetime: back pain? Lifted-heel footwear props our body forward, and thus our low back becomes excessively curved to pull us back into alignment. This ripple of tension weasels its way up to the cervical spine (neck) to compensate for the newfound tension down the chain, leading to the fairly ubiquitous complaint of a "tight" neck. Contrary to the popular kids' song, the ankle bone is actually connected to every other bone in the body, and its movement is associated with your production of neurochemistry (although for the sake of singing in class, it'd be sensible to stick the original version).

Preventing the heel from fully dropping as it would on any natural surface in bare feet adds a new variable of tension to the body that modern humans are struggling to cope with. A body held in this tensed and imbalanced position becomes a ticking time bomb waiting for some part to "pop" along the postural chain at a seemingly random moment. Was that pillow you were picking up extra heavy when you threw your back out that day, or have you been setting the stage for the injury to transpire for years with improper footwear and imbalanced movement patterns?

FUN FACT

1-inch heels add 22 percent more pressure on the forefoot.
2-inch heels add 57 percent.
3-inch heels add 76 percent.

I would venture to say the physically deleterious effect of consistent high heel use (key word here is "consistent"—occasional use is no problem, as far as I can tell) is at least on par with that of the neck-lengthening traditions practiced in Asia we as foreigners would typically find to be outlandish. There, I said it. The good news is we can begin decompressing and unwinding our postural imbalances via self-care, better movement choices, and proper footwear.

A BRIEF HISTORY OF HEELS

For the record, high heels are not some newfangled thing, but have been used as tools for literally thousands of years. Their functions have ranged from lifting ancient Egyptian butchers' feet off the ground to avoid standing in the blood of animals, to a war tool for Persian soldiers on horseback to secure their feet in the stirrups while standing to shoot a bow, to elevating European aristocrats off the ground to avoid stepping in horse crap and to appear taller to denote more authority. In fact, the red high heel wasn't popularized by the likes of Christian Louboutin, but originally were worn by men in the French court during the seventeenth century. King Louis XIV used red heels as an indication of those in royal favor, and no one could wear heels taller than his, which measured a whopping five inches tall! This all lasted until the great male renunciation, when male style shifted away from adornment and beauty toward utility.

I've included this brief, slightly ridiculous history of heels mainly because I found it super interesting. I'm not here to rain on anyone's heel parade—I just want all the well-meaning people using them as the tool they are to know the risks of excessive use. If you've insulated yourself with enough healthy self-care and functional movement in other aspects of your life, I don't see a problem with wearing heels for short periods of time (like less than an hour). That wasn't easy for me to write, but I think the heel lovers out there needed to hear it, and we'll both feel a lot better now that I've said it.

ALIGN YOUR SHIRTS: THE HANG TEST

Remember the squat test for your pants? This is like that but for your shirts. When buying a shirt or jacket (gentlemen) or any kind of women's wear (ladies), reach up to touch a doorway to be sure the sleeves move with ease. If your clothing limits you in any way, you are setting yourself up for inflexibility and an aversion to play because you don't want to rip your new article of what is hopefully organic fabric.

That's right, organic fabric! Your skin absorbs the dyes and various chemicals used to create your clothing. The underlying costs of fast fashion are a topic for another book, but I implore you to take a deeper look into where your clothing comes from and choose companies based on their global impact whenever possible.

RETHINK YOUR FASHION

Footwear

- Wide toe box (should not crowd or compress your feet at all)

- Flats (it may take time to adapt to zero-drop shoes; take it slowly if you're accustomed to more heel support)

- Flexible (can you roll them up?)

Pants and shorts

- Can you squat in them with full range of motion?

- Organic materials whenever possible

Shirts

- Can you hang in them?

- Organic materials whenever possible

Underwear

- Loose-fitting or supportive without restricting motion and/or bloodflow

- Organic materials whenever possible

- For men: Banana hammocks are appropriate only on special occasions

Alignment Assignment

I can hear critics stirring at the idea of converting to more minimalist footwear—this journey is not for the faint of heart. It's a gradual process that takes time, and most people get themselves into trouble by jumping straight to minimalist shoes without foot training prior. Here's a simple recipe to help rehabilitate domesticated feet.

1. Stand with your feet placed under your sit bones more often. Stacking your feet under your pelvic bones (ischial tuberosities) while standing will help naturally re-form the foot architecture to be more support- ive instead of the collapsed pattern typical with many people. As you're standing, you can alternate between gripping the ground with your toes and spreading them wide and lifting them off the ground for ten or so repetitions.

2. Barefoot practice on sand, rocks, logs, etc.

3. Take it slowly: Hang on to your old shoes, and split time between your old and new ones until your feet are strong enough to drop the support completely.

4. Tippy-toe walks: This is a great (and fun) way to re-strengthen your arches while working on balance at the same time. Focus on all the principles for aligned standing outlined in Chapter 6 while you raise yourself up on your tippy-toes. Emphasize the weight on the first and

second toe, but feel all five firmly grounded to feel stable. You can raise your arms overhead and/or walk forward and backward for six steps, and remember to breathe!

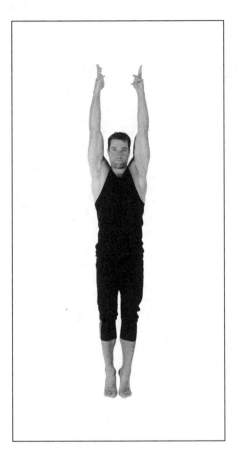

CHAPTER 10

Align Your Home for Optimal Health and Creativity

"We shape our buildings and afterwards our buildings shape us."

—*Winston Churchill*

Have you ever noticed the way a room makes you feel? The colors, placement of furniture (or lack thereof), lighting, windows, art, instruments, and old family photos can all create a distinctive sensation.

A variety of studies show our physical environment has a large impact on mood and mental well-being.[1] Did you know, for example, that the room in which you're presently sitting is being mapped within the hippocampus of your brain? That's right, you are literally being neurologically imprinted as we speak—the room is becoming a part of you. As humans, we have an immense capacity for adaptation. We can't help but become formed by not just the people we spend time with, the books we read, and the food we eat, but also the physical spaces and environments we occupy. Pay attention to how you keep your home, as it stays within your cortical maps even after you walk out the door. On top of the brain being imprinted by the rooms in which we reside, cellular biologists have shown we are changed all way down to the cellular level by the way we experience our environment.[2]

Dr. Sergio Altomonte, architect and associate professor in the Department of Architecture and Built Environment at Nottingham University in England, said, "Buildings and urban spaces should be designed first and foremost around their occupants. The importance of architecture as a trigger to physical, physiological and psychological well-being is nowadays becoming a topic of significant relevance."[3] This is especially important considering modern Americans spend upwards of 90 percent of their time indoors!

Most of us will never design a building or city impacting thousands of people each day, but we can engineer our own home to cultivate mental, physical, and emotional success for whoever occupies the space. This is one of the best gifts you can offer your own life and the lives of your children, who are far more affected by what you do and the manner in which you keep your home than by what you say. Every time you walk through the door, your subconscious mind is determining if the place feels safe, creative, balanced, strong, and vibrant or closed, disorganized, unstable, dark, and insecure. This is a survival mechanism that has helped our species perpetuate itself for millennia—it's kind of a big deal. Let's get started forming your home for optimal health and get this self-preserving feedback loop working in your favor!

SIMPLE STEPS TO ALIGN YOUR "LIVING" ROOM

"A house is a home when it shelters the body and comforts the soul."
—*Phillip Moffitt*

Step 1: Floor Cushions and Comfy Rugs

Your body becomes structurally molded by the chair you sit on, similar to the way we imprint our butts on the chair itself. As we've discussed earlier, the first thing to do when aligning your home is to get low. Make the floor of your home more inviting by softening it up. Comfortable rugs, floor pillows, cushions, yoga mats, etc., will subconsciously invite you and your company to journey toward the ground more often.

If you want to impress your New Age friends and make the ground even more therapeutic, I personally use a BioMat for a bit of infrared heat therapy.

Step 2: Add Self-Care Tools

Most of us are naturally opportunistic: We will do the thing in front of us and forget what's not in sight. So put the things that make you and your family healthier in your visual field. As discussed in Chapter 7, throw a pull-up bar in a doorway you walk through regularly, and every time you pass through, knock out a couple of reps or get in a shoulder-saving hang. Now that you are spending more time on the floor, toss a couple different size balls, a foam roller, and a resistance band on the ground to add some myofascial release to your computer or TV time.

I have an Align Band hanging from a closet door at my house specifically so it's in my visual field (for those in long-distance relationships, perhaps cover your eyes for this next sentence). What's not in sight will likely be forgotten, so put the things that provide you the most growth in your daily walking path around the house, office, or wherever you spend a lot of time. By the same token, remove the stuff that wastes your time or diverts your attention from your priorities (chairs that put you in a dysfunctional position, junk food in your pantry, digital distractions).

Making the right decision becomes easy when you organize your environment for healthy choices to be in your visual field, giving them a place at the top of your mind. Your home, office, and travel environments are like hands molding clay on a pottery wheel, and you're the pot—it's wise to pay attention while the wheel is spinning (the wheel is always spinning).

STEP 3: MAKE ART INTERACTIVE

"Art lives where absolute freedom is, because where it is not, there can be no creativity."

—*Bruce Lee*

Instruments serve as an excellent form of interactive art, because even when they aren't being played, they're beautiful and filled with meaning. Start incorporating interactive art into your home (and actually interact with it). Get yourself a dry-erase or chalk board and regularly switch out inspiring quotes or scribble a new doodle on the board to match your mood. You can even buy paint that turns an entire section of a wall into a canvas to scribble on. (I did this in my home and people love it!) If something doesn't feel worth interacting with in your home, it's likely time to let it go.

Your residence is an outward projection of your mind, and the most important part of a happy home is a happy mind. It's a bit like a Russian doll set, in which each layer mimics the next. Your own personal Russian doll sequence may look like this: The innermost spiritual layer is followed by the emotional layer, mental layer, home layer, proximal community layer, state, country, globe, and as far out as you would like to extrapolate. Each form affects the next on either side, and any impact on one will trickle into the rest. This may be what Gandhi meant when he suggested, "You must be the change you want to see in the world."

MAKE A NAP NOOK

Hold on, I thought this book was about movement and posture, you may be thinking. Well, if you're tired, good luck standing upright and appearing energetic. Your posture is a representation of how you feel. If you're often exhausted, you'll tend to slouch, which in turn makes you feel even more tired, forming a hazardous feedback loop. Our connective tissue forms to whatever position we are regularly in, for good or ill. If you feel drained and tired due to imbalanced sleep patterns, there is no lacrosse ball, foam roller, resistance band, or supplement on this planet that will get you to stand upright, move energetically, and shine. Healthy sleep (and diet) could be likened to the raw materials it takes to form an "aligned" physical structure. If you're tired, go take a nap—it may be just the postural boost you've been looking for.

Earlier today, I jumped into a cold plunge (information on how to create your own can be found at TheAlignBook.com) with a good buddy, Colin Wilson, who plays professional ice hockey for the Colorado Avalanche. For him or any professional athlete, it's invaluable to analyze each detail of their day and night, in search of any potential performance boosts. As we were chatting about some of these details, Colin passively dropped some sage advice I'll never forget: "Sleep is a weapon." We undervalue the potential of a good nap as we trudge through the day's work, but studies show taking a simple ten- to twenty-minute siesta will boost alertness, enhance mood, and increase memory retention. And many cultures around the world often take a snooze break in the afternoon because there's a small increase in body temperature between one and three p.m., which releases snooze-promoting melatonin. The return on investment from a quick power nap is unlike any supplement you could ever purchase. No wonder Google and other tech companies have installed nap pods in their offices.

Like anything else, studies show timing is a key ingredient to make your midday shut-eye most effective. Ideally, shoot for a nap time of under thirty minutes, or go all out for a full ninety minutes. A brief nap will keep you in the lighter stages of non-rapid-eye-movement (NREM) sleep. If you enter into the deeper stages of sleep and then have to abruptly wake up, you will notice a groggier sensation upon rising commonly referred to as "sleep inertia," instead of the energy boost you're looking for to enhance your performance at work. Timing is key to stay on the opposite side of sleep inertia.

If you have the time and need to pay off some lingering sleep debt from the previous night, go all out for a full ninety-minute nap to allow your body go through a full sleep cycle. It seemed to work well for leaders like JFK and

Winston Churchill. A full sleep cycle allows your body to wake up more easily and is associated with boosting creativity, enhancing procedural memory (motor skills such as driving, walking, or riding a bike), and elevating emotional memory (recalling events, people, or situations).[4]

One last bit on timing. Psychology professor and nap researcher Sara Mednick, PhD, suggests that there are more and less optimal times of day to nap, depending upon when you wake up in the morning. For example, an early riser who usually gets up at five a.m. will get the most value of napping around one p.m., whereas a night owl getting up around nine a.m. will derive more benefit from a siesta closer to three p.m. This and more is detailed in her book, *Take a Nap!*[5]

ALIGN YOUR TOILET

It would be pretty *assi*nine (get it?) for me to discuss how to align your home and leave out the holy grail. I'm just going to say it: Your body is designed (since the beginning of humanity) for you to defecate on flat ground, which involves squatting deeper than ninety degrees. You can get fairly close to replicating the position by simply raising your legs up on some type of stool placed in front of a Western style raised toilet. (Squatty Potty is a popular choice for a pooping stool.)

Why does this matter, you ask? While in a standing or sitting position your rectum is in its "closed for business" position, meaning the puborectalis muscle is tugging the rectum, which essentially kinks the hose at an angle to maintain continence. When you go into a squat position, this angle (referred to as the anorectal angle) opens up to unkink the "hose" and allow for an easy and healthy defecation. If you are a person who is pushing and reading a magazine on the toilet, you have some work to do. A healthy poop should take mere seconds, and raising your knees up while you go will make for a healthier colon and assist in relieving unnecessary pushing, leading to sub-optimal experiences such as hemorrhoids.

Alignment Assignment

Here are a couple must-have Align Band exercises you can do in your home after spending time typing on a computer or if you regularly use a cell phone.

Shoulder Decompression

Set the band at shoulder height and pass the loop around the targeted shoulder. Face away from the door in a lunge position and walk yourself away from the

door to put a stretch on the shoulder, pulling it posteriorly. Hinge your hips forward to create a downward pull on the shoulder to decompress the neck muscles as well. Reach your fingertips down to the ground and then begin raising them with your arm up above your head to help mobilize the shoulder joint. Be explorative with this movement, and feel free take each arm through any variety of movements that feel helpful in relaxing the tense tissues. Work with each shoulder for about ninety seconds, and remember to breathe.

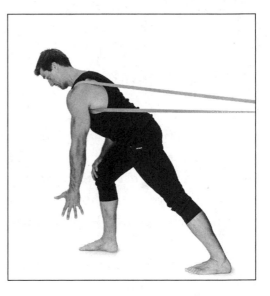

Neck Decompression

This may be my favorite technique for reversing the unsightly pattern of forward head posture. Place the band at the top of the door so that it's hanging down the middle from a height above your head. Facing the door, place the loop of the band behind your neck at the base of your skull just above or on top of your ears and inch yourself backward to create a lifting and decompression of the cervical spine (neck). Pull your chin and head back to lengthen the neck and activate the muscles in the back. Hold this contraction for about thirty to sixty seconds. Repeat two to three times, and notice how much taller you feel afterward!

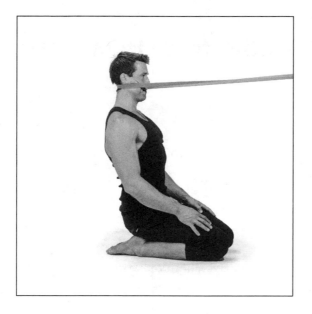

CHAPTER 11

Aligning Your Office for Better Movement

"How we spend our days is, of course, how we spend our lives."

—*Annie Dillard*

The average American spends 8.7 hours at work on the average workday, according the aptly named American Time Use Survey. Those precious hours in your office add up to about fourteen years and four months of your life at work![1] If how we spend our days is truly how we spend our life, it would make sense to dial in our office experience so it's something we can look back at and say, "Heck yeah, I spent fourteen years in my office—it was the best room in the house!"

We largely still accept an antiquated story of how the office is supposed to look. An artificially lit room with a thermostat preventing your body from doing any pesky temperature regulation along with a large desk with sharp corners and lots of space for us to sign important documents, a prestigious leather chair, a few paperweights, and perhaps a trophy buck on the wall to remind you that you're the man (or woman) of the space. This traditional office model is fighting to hang on, but I think it's about time to put it to rest for good.

I should note, there's another model that's becoming increasingly popular, as well: the open floor plan. The stereotype here is a giant, wall-less room filled with long rows of dozens of employees working at their computer stations, most of whom have headphones on to cut themselves off from each other. More likely than not, though, the basic setup is still chair, screen, keyboard—just out in the open. This is a step in the right direction, but could still use a lot of improvement if the goal is healthy bodies and productive minds for employees.

We really should look on the bright side, though: The old model of extended chair sitting has served back surgeons very well. We spend approximately $90 billion annually on the diagnosis and management of low-back pain.[2] Before we start making any rash decisions around enriching modern work environments with movement opportunities to heal the spines of employed people, let's be respectful and take a moment of silence for the spine docs out there who might miss a yacht payment. All right, moment taken—let's heal some backs!

STANDING DESK, FLOOR DESK, OR BOTH?

Sorry to break the news to you, but there is no one magic bullet position or posture that will save the world or your body. Standing desks have become misunderstood as a panacea for improving health in the workplace. The reality is that standing is just another range of motion; if done excessively, it brings a similar set of problems to the ones we were attempting to avoid with chair sitting. It should be known that the standing, or tadasana (mountain), pose in yoga is an incredibly technical position, and the value you derive from your standing desk is directly influenced by the quality of your standing mechanics.

The keys to a pain-free, flexible, and healthy body are continual postural shifts in a variety of balanced ranges of motion. If you can, I *highly* recommend embracing the floor culture concept discussed previously in your daily work life if it's possible in your occupation (tag #floorculture to share your setup with the Align Community!). For those that are bound to a traditional desk to pay the bills, what follows are a few key points to optimize your movement.

Raise Your Screen Height

If your screen is low, there's a good chance you're practicing a postural state of depression (Mopey archetype) while at work. An aligned, upright position is linked to uplifting one's mood and confidence, while the inverse is true with a slumped-over position. Get yourself into your most upright sitting or standing (if you have a standing desk) position and align the screen to the height of your head or even slightly above to encourage even more growth (most people literally will grow taller as they begin aligning their posture). This will be a friendly reminder to continually return your body to an upright, stacked position and start to retrain your eyes to look up instead of being glued to the ground.

Keep Your Pelvis above the Knees

If you are sitting on a chair, refer back to the principles discussed in Chapter 6—it's your blueprint for sitting on a chair from now on. The starting point to sit functionally on a chair is to make sure your pelvis is raised above your knees, as this puts your pelvis and low back in a more balanced position by allowing you to rest on the front edge of your sit bones (ischial tuberosities).

What does it mean for your low back and pelvis to be in a more balanced position? you may ask. As we learned previously, your lowest vertebrae are actually a bit more wedge-shaped, naturally tilting your pelvis forward just a bit in a sitting position. You want to embrace that curve in the sitting position, and the seat height is a crucial part of making that happen. This will save your lumbar discs from being squished continuously throughout the workday, setting you up for a long and healthy relationship with your spine.

Eye Breaks—Get a Window

A frequently cited study published in 1984 in the *Journal of Science* by environmental psychologist Roger Ulrich showed the powerful healing effects of placing post-surgery patients by a bedside window exposed to leafy trees, compared to a brick wall. Patients with a view healed and were ready to be released from the hospital a full day faster on average, used less pain medication, and experienced fewer post-surgical complications.[3]

If you are calm, content, and living in a more parasympathetic state during your workday, you will be more productive, happier, and healthier. If relocating your office to a room with a window is not possible, make regular trips outside to recharge (or, perhaps think about changing careers). At a bare minimum, every twenty minutes or so, take an "eye break" to look to points at various distances from you to exercise your eye muscles' full range of motion. For more on this, check out Chapter 15.

Switch Hands Regularly

Would you like to boost creativity at work while preventing wrist pain? An interesting study published in the *Journal of Experimental Psychology: General* by Dr. Michael Slepian and fellow researchers found those who drew fluid lines on a computer screen with their finger, versus rigid, straight lines, experienced an increase in divergent thinking skills.[4] After several repetitions of drawing these sketches, the fluid movement group experienced measurably greater creativity and cognitive flexibility. This creative ability was determined by how these fluid-drawing subjects solved problems, recommended solutions, and made abstract associations in a more creative way than their more rigid controls.

Now, while you're at it, try compounding the fluidity of your movement by more regularly using your less dominant hand! Wrist problems have become far too common in our modern world, and repetitive stress is a major culprit. These issues can be alleviated and/or prevented entirely by expanding the range of motion on both sides of your body. Regularly add a few minutes of clicking on your computer mouse or scrolling on your phone with your non-dominant hand. By noticing how much you do with your dominant hand and making a conscious effort to make the movement fluid, which represents effective motor control, your brain and body will thank you!

Tight wrists? Try this band exercise to decompress your wrists and shoulders after working too long on a computer.

Hand Decompression

Set the Align Band up at shoulder height and place one hand at the end of the band. Open your hand wide so the band catches the edge of your palm and walk away from the door to put a stretch into the band and your shoulder and wrist. Stand tall and reach your arm out while the band provides traction on your wrist and shoulder to unwind the stress of repetitive typing or screen scrolling. Hold this stretch for about sixty seconds on each arm (or whatever feels best for you), and remember to breathe calmly, emphasizing the exhale.

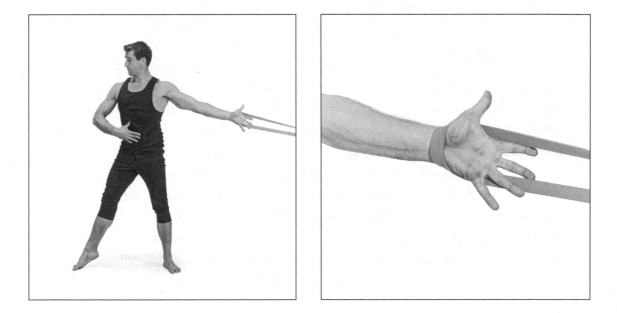

THE HEALTH BENEFITS OF INCONVENIENCE

Let's be honest, working out to stay in shape is fairly inconvenient. So are cold showers, going to a store to buy flowers for a loved one, planting a garden, traveling to arrive at the most gorgeous place you've ever seen, etc. It's embracing these inconveniences of life that grants us permission to arrive at a more desirable destination fit only for those willing to put in the work to get there. We often outsource the inconvenience of simple daily movements—such as having groceries delivered so you don't have to walk around the grocery store, using a button to open the trunk of your car instead of pulling it open with your hands, or raising your furniture to a height such that you never actually need to bend your hips below ninety degrees in any given day. The movement Western culture has done such a good job at trimming out of daily life is exactly what we've evolved over millennia to do, and is paramount to the workings of your physiology. We now need to supplement with obscure workouts, mainly because our daily life has been stripped of its nourishing movement variables.[5]

There is power in doing things the "long, hard, stupid way," as celebrated restaurateur and proprietor of the famed Momofuku restaurant chain David Chang has suggested. Take your time to support the health of your mind and body while you're there. You get out exactly what you put in, no more, no less—if you can find joy in the journey, life becomes a breeze.

What a person deems convenient or inconvenient is more about mind-set than the action itself. You can alter your mind to take pleasure in movement by gradually incorporating a few healthy "inconveniences" into your workday, and you'll find they actually end up saving you time because you'll have more energy and concentration when you go back to work. Creating more reasons to get up and take a walk during your workday, no matter how brief, instead of "efficiently" remaining seated and having the world come to you is a key to longevity, healthy body composition, and brain health. In a past Align Podcast interview, Dr. Kelly Starrett gave a simple example of how to add more health-inducing "inconvenience" to your home or office by using one common trash can in the house, causing you to naturally add extra steps to your day. Another option would be to leave your cell phone away from your working area so that each time you need to use it requires getting up for a brief walk. Such small daily steps multiplied over a year come out to some serious mileage, translating to calories burned, fat metabolized, and muscle gained. As Kelly often says, "Be consistent, then we can talk about being heroic."

Joan Vernikos, former director of NASA's Life Sciences Division, suggests that our bodies function optimally on continuous low-intensity movements (such as regularly getting up and down from the ground or adding more walking time to your day) instead of the breakneck transition of a predominantly sedentary day followed by a blow-out CrossFit or Soul Cycle class to make up for lost time. Simple household tasks or movement around your office, if done regularly and with care and efficient mechanics, aggregate to sustained structural change and increased energy levels with time. The key is to optimize your movement throughout the whole day.

THE PLAYFUL WORKPLACE

> "It is not uncommon for people to spend their whole life waiting to start living."
>
> —*Eckhart Tolle*

A lot of tech companies looking to attract talented millennials are no longer focusing on only dangling high starting salaries and competitive benefits. They're also putting in pool, air hockey, and Ping-Pong tables, laying dodgeball courts, and even building in slides that employees can use to access lower levels instead of taking the stairs. On the surface, these perks might seem like recruiting gimmicks, yet what the leaders of these companies may or may not realize is that in addition to creating a cool culture, they're also enhancing employee performance.

"At work, play has been found to speed up learning, enhance productivity and increase job satisfaction," Lynn Barnett, a professor of recreation, sports, and tourism at the University of Illinois at Urbana-Champaign, told the *Washington Post*.[6]

If you're a manager or executive, consider how you can foster playfulness in the workplace. You don't need to try and compete with the Googles and Facebooks of your industry—simply grabbing a dartboard or bringing in movement classes during lunchtime would make a massive difference. Not at the decision-making level? Then go to your boss and suggest ways to bring more movement and play to the office, and explain the research behind it. She will likely appreciate the idea to spark more life to the company. If she rebuts your case, you can give her a copy of this book to explain why it matters (shameless promotion, I realize).

ADDING EXTRA GRAVITY TO YOUR OFFICE—REBOUNDER

I'll be honest, when I first heard of people using these in their offices, I found it to be cute at best. It wasn't until I tried a good one at Aubrey Marcus's office at Onnit HQ in Austin that I completely changed my tune. A trampoline of any sort is one incredible way to increase G-forces on the body in a joint-friendly and fun manner. Running will certainly do so, but the sad reality is few modern deskbound bodies are adequately structured to run without exacerbating pre-existing joint issues. Don't get me wrong, running is a spectacular movement practice, but most adults just need to be retrained on how to run effectively, so their knees don't catch fire and hips tighten up even more than all that sitting has already encouraged.

Astronauts returning home from space are found to have essentially experienced the effects of rapid aging during their gravity sabbatical. The lack of gravity sets the stage for rapid reduction in bone density, for example. On Earth, people tend to lose about 1 percent of their bone density per year after the age of twenty. Remove the continuous pressure of gravity and that number goes to about 1.6 percent per month and has been reported to be as much as 1 percent loss in a week! Joan Vernikos found the closest way to replicate the rapid aging effects of anti-gravity is to study subjects continuously lying down, because the gravitational pull is distributed across subjects' bodies instead of pulling down-ward from head to toe. This is the magic of rebounding—you are stacking the body upright and piling healing G-forces through your structure repeatedly, all while smiling and taking yourself less seriously. (It's very hard to play serious tough guy on a four-foot-wide trampoline, trust me on this.)

Regular rebounding will also circulate the clear, colorless fluid called lymph that's responsible for flushing toxins from your body, in turn supporting your immune system and overall physiological well-being.[7] Using a mini trampo-line regularly has been shown to increase balance, strength, and proprioception, which is our ability to sense the orientation, position, and movement of the body and its parts. It took some time to win me over, but I've come around, and a rebounder in your office is Align approved. If you don't have access to a rebounder, any form of jumping around will do the trick but will not be nearly as fun as a mini trampoline in your office. Happy bouncing!

Alignment Assignment

If you do any work from a laptop, bring it to the ground by placing your com-puter on a low table, chair, couch, or on the floor. Grab some cushions to raise your butt up while you sit for comfort and to put your spine into a more aligned position. Be sure to alternate sitting positions every ten or so minutes to keep your body moving while you work. If working from the ground is not an option, get yourself a chair large enough so you can cross your legs and throw a cushion under your butt to raise your hips as though you're sitting on the floor.

If you are using a standing desk, try this technique to work on your Aligned Standing position: Start by spreading your toes open wide and imagine your big toe, pinky toe, and both sides of your heels are being subtly pulled in all four directions. Then imagine you have a magnetic pull tugging your big toe to the inside of your heel and pinky toe to the outside of your heel, activating both medial (inside) and lateral (outside) arches of the foot.

Alternate between lifting all your toes from the ground as high as you can and grasping them against the ground, while maintaining solid contact with all four "corners" of the feet. If this feels easy, play with doing so while standing on one foot at a time, by subtly plugging your standing leg into the ground, elongating from the hip, and causing the opposite side leg to lift slightly (imagine you're growing your femur out from the hip socket). It's a great, discreet way to work on your own self-care in public without being "that guy" doing downward facing dogs in the middle of a wedding.

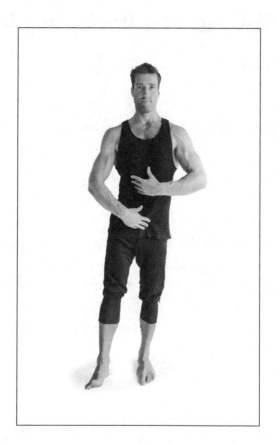

CHAPTER 12

Therapeutic Movement for Driving and Travel

"Those who do not move do not notice their chains."

—Rosa Luxemburg

It's entirely too easy to use travel as an excuse for not taking adequate care of your body. The reality is most car, plane, train, or bus seats holding your butt in place are inherently dysfunctional for your physical structure and overall well-being. It's OK. There's hope! There are some body-saving travel fundamentals you can incorporate into any commute, flight, or random hotel which quite literally will save your butt.

CAR TIME

To say Americans spend a lot of time in the car is a vast understatement. The AAA Foundation averaged this to be around 290 hours each year! That's over twelve full days hunkered behind the wheel. If you spent 290 hours each year practicing anything, you'd eventually become pretty good at it.[1] The problem with dedicating all those hours to driving is that in this case, practice doesn't make perfect, it simply reinforces imbalanced patterns. Car seats form the body into the archetypal structural positions of feeling down or defensive, as we discussed in the first chapter. The head juts forward, the shoulder and spine roll forward, the tail tucks under like a scared dog, and the legs are fairly disengaged for most of the car ride, unless you drive a stick shift. That's 17,600 minutes forcing you to practice the structural position of depression. I wonder if this could affect the way a person feels (sarcasm).

It's no wonder longer commute times have been associated with increased risk of physical and emotional disorder! Researchers from the Washington University School of Medicine in Saint Louis and the Cooper Institute in Dallas found people with commutes of at least ten miles each way to be more likely to experience anxiety, depression, and social isolation.[2] That's not to mention the spike in blood pressure, rise in blood sugar, and the sore back and neck you may get prior to walking into your big business meeting. A study from the United Kingdom's Office of National Statistics made the connection that longer commute times are associated with lower life satisfaction and decreased feelings of happiness.[3]

It's fairly simple math; your body forms to the positions in which you spend the most time, and that affects your health and happiness. We spend heaps of time transporting ourselves from place to place and thus will adapt to the form of our transportation. We can do better, and it's a fairly simple fix with some basic tips!

Water Break

It's always a good idea to travel with a water bottle, but not just to stay hydrated. It can double as a spine mobilizer and alignment device. Place the bottle vertically or horizontally (a pillow or cushion may be more comfortable for the uninitiated) around your mid back and practice breathing into the area when you're driving (obviously stay focused on the road as you're doing so). This props your spine up into a stronger and more neutral position instead of the sad-shrimp spine shape car seats and sofas push us into.

Raise the Mirrors in Your Car

Next time you get into your car, sit up into a tall, confident posture (it will help if you're using a pillow or bottle behind your back to effortlessly support the position) and adjust your mirrors to fit the taller version of yourself. It will act as a subtle reminder each time you check your mirror to create some length in your spine. This is a simple hack you can implement in your driving to start, but please keep this idea in mind in other places as well. For example, start placing items in higher places in your cabinets so you have to reach up on a more regular basis to mobilize your shoulders, increase lung capacity, and encourage your eye muscles to look up. Think of your body as a plant growing toward the sun and bending its shape along the way; you'll bend and pattern to the shape of your environment in a similar way!

Squeeze!

The major issue with driving is the prolonged passivity of your body, which inevitably causes fluids you want to circulate to stagnate instead. The other big problem with driving is the sub-optimal position your body is being trained into (because training extends beyond the gym, remember?). It's of paramount importance you organize your body into a more upright position while you practice the isometric exercises I'm about to discuss. Start by stacking your spine in a more neutral position with a cushion, bottle, small roller, or something of the sort as discussed in the last section, and then you can use the door, your own knees, the steering wheel, your seat, and literally anything you come in contact with as your "exercise equipment."

I first discovered isometric training when I was a teenager, via old Bruce Lee books, and it's stuck with me ever since. This approach was a staple for his strength training, and you have an amazing opportunity to practice the same thing while driving! There are essentially three basic types of muscular contraction you can practice: concentric, eccentric, and isometric. Concentric is the shortening of muscle tissue, eccentric is the lengthening, and isometric is contracting from a static position. A study done in 2001 measured these three types of muscular contraction and found the isometric contraction to produce the greatest activation of the muscles, not to mention it can be done in tight places like a car . . .

The study stated, "The mean activation levels during maximal eccentric and maximal concentric contractions were 88.3% and 89.7%, respectively, and were significantly lower with respect to maximal isometric contractions (95.2%)."[4] This can lead to serious strength gains if that's what you're seeking, or it can just be a great way to tone your muscles and assist with circulation while you're cooped up for your commute! I know what you're likely thinking: "That's great information, but what the heck does that have to do with being in the car?"

If you want to follow in Bruce Lee's footsteps (that's pretty much all of us, right?), you can hold your isometric contractions for six to twelve seconds at a maximum effort; since safety is the most important thing, treat this more as a tissue massage than a workout and take it easy. Please don't attempt to rip your steering wheel off and blame me for it. Use your discretion while tinkering with all this. The main point of these techniques is to circulate blood and lymphatic fluid while creating some muscular tone as an added benefit.

ISOMETRIC CAR TECHNIQUES

Disclaimer: Practice these techniques while your car is stopped.

For each of these techniques, hold the contraction at around 30 percent to 40 percent (or whatever feels comfortable and safe) for five to eight seconds and repeat at each stoplight or whatever feels best for you. Remember to comfortably breathe through your nose as you're engaging your muscles.

Glute Press

Butt falling asleep? Reclaim your butt muscles by engaging them while you're on a road trip. Simply press your heels down into the floor until you feel your butt muscles activate and hold for five to eight seconds.

Hip Abduction

Reactivate the "side butt" by pressing your knees outward against the side of your door and the center column.

Hip Adduction

Turn on the muscles on the inside of your legs by simply pressing your knees together. You will feel your adductor muscles engage and perhaps even feel the muscles of the pelvic floor.

Steering Wheel Sequence (Medial/External Rotation, Protraction/Retraction)

This sequence of techniques is invaluable for the health of your shoulder girdles while driving. Simply grasp the steering wheel at around nine and three o'clock, then alternate between rotating your wrists outward and then inward to start. You can then alternate between pulling and pushing the steering wheel toward and away from you.

Spine Extension

Does your back feel tight? Often, the feelings of tension are not because the muscles are locked in a short position, but instead they are locked long from chronically being hunched forward in chairs. You can help rebalance these muscles by pressing your head, shoulders, and upper back against the car seat like you are retracting into a back-extension machine in a gym.

Ab Curl (Bracing Hands against the Wheel)

Tone your abs and assist in organ function by bracing your hands against the steering wheel and contracting your abs by pushing your upper body forward against the pressure of your hands on the wheel.

SQUAT AND LUNGE BREAK

"Before beginning a program of physical inactivity, see your doctor. Sedentary living is abnormal and dangerous to your health."

—*Frank Forencich*

The squat is arguably the mother of the functional movement family to maintain longevity and overall health. Squatting acts as a pressure release for your hips and organs and is crucially important for blood and lymphatic circulation through your lower body. The lunge is equally important because it more closely resembles walking, running, and a variety of movement patterns. This motion creates a rotational force on the organs a bit like that of twisting a rag to squeeze out fluid held within the fabric. This motion is your body's natural fluid pump and visceral massage system at work. Every time you perform these motions, you're turning on the pump to clean your system. If you were a pond, suppose you would require a 1,000-gallon-per-hour pump to circulate your water in order for it to remain optimally healthy and the aquatic creatures to thrive.

Now imagine what would happen to that pond if you decided to skimp with a 300-gallon-per-hour pump, and only circulated the water in certain parts; this would spell trouble for the health and homeostasis of your ecosystem. Your body is an ecosystem much like the pond and requires adequate circulation in the form of regular movement to thrive.

Think about this each time you're on a road trip. Taking a break every hour or so for a brisk walk, five or six lunges, and a few squats is all it takes to turn your internal pumping system back on after the arduous journey of extended chair sitting.

Squat with Align Band

Wrapping a resistance band around your knees as you're squatting is a great way to help engage your gluteal (aka butt) muscles during the motion. Be sure to keep heavy contact with your big toes on the ground as you push your knees outward against the band. Follow the same principles outlined in Chapter 6 as you go through the squatting motion.

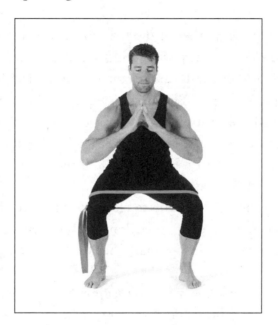

Crescent Lunge

This is a staple motion to practice and a great way to unwind from the stress and tension of travel. Step with one leg in front of you a few feet or so from the back foot, and keep both feet pointing straight ahead as though you're on railroad tracks. Keep strong contact with all four corners of your feet and begin to lower your hips, while raising your back heel off the ground. Imagine there is pole behind your back that you're sliding yourself down so your spine stays completely neutral through the whole movement.

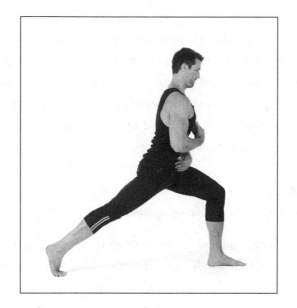

ALIGN YOURSELF

For each hour of sitting on a road trip, take at least five minutes to pull over for some muscular activation and joint mobilization. Try taking a brisk walk and include five lunges on each leg, five air squats, and get your arms up overhead by finding something to hang on to or simply extending your arms overhead while you're lunging (visit TheAlignBook .com for video guides on road trip mobility). If you dare, toss a skateboard or pair of roller skates (it's time to bring back the eighties!) in your trunk to add a dose of balance, play, and an extra form of transportation when you arrive at your destination.

AIRPLANE MODE

Airplane mode should be a very commonly used feature on every phone. There aren't too many sensible reasons I can think of to have your cell phone emitting radiation from your pocket beside your sexual organs all day long. It's even worse inside your car, because the radiation from your cell phone is reflected back to you by the metallic structure of the car. This magnifies the radiation to you and your fellow passengers' bodies. I personally keep my phone on airplane mode anytime it's in my pocket (every now and again, I forget, it's OK) and will take it off only when I need a signal, which is surpassingly rare if you take a few steps:

- Download podcasts, music, audiobooks, etc., instead of streaming, so airplane mode is an option while using media.

- Use headphones or speaker phone instead of putting the phone directly up to your face (avoid holding the phone while it's off airplane mode when you can).

- You can change the color of your screen to be grayscale, which reduces the addictive effects of screen staring. We love to see colors, and when the screen isn't popping with them, it's less interesting to pick up.

AIRPLANE TRAVEL

Traveling can add a lot of stress to your life and body, especially if you're going long distances crammed into uncomfortable positions. In addition to the exercises in this chapter, I'm also sharing some of my favorite methods to actively remind my body to relax so the tension of a long TSA line doesn't live in my shoulders for hours.

This is one of the more challenging nuts to crack in the travel self-care equation, but it's doable. Spending a lot of time hunkered down in an airplane while being shuffled through a gross airport with enough radiation to pop corn is tough on the body, but there are some fundamental travel hacks that will make your travel time more healthy and pleasurable.

Compression Socks

Compression stockings are a hot topic in the running community, being touted to help with endurance and reduce muscular soreness from distance running. This is by no means a new phenomenon. The usage of compression therapy is mentioned in the Edwin Smith Papyrus, the oldest known surgical document, discovered in Egypt and dating back to the seventeenth century B.C.; and they're mentioned again by Hippocrates, who wrote about using them to prevent blood from pooling in the legs with patients in the fourth century B.C.[5]

Compression can assist with circulation, decrease leg swelling during travel, improve symptoms of vein disease, and assist with the prevention of blood clots. A deep vein thrombosis (DVT) is a blood clot that forms in one of your major veins deep inside your body. This affects as many as 900,000 people annually, and up to 100,000 people lose their lives from the condition.[6] Your circulation is no joke, and the use of compression therapy while sitting for extended periods can help.

Walk the Halls

As discussed previously, walking is your best (and least silly looking) ally for optimizing fluid circulation while flying. Follow the same formula as for driving: For each hour of sitting while flying, be sure to get in at least five minutes of walking. It's optimal to incorporate this formula hourly instead of back- or front-loading the walking time. Embrace being *that* guy or girl who is busting out a few lunges or squats by the bathroom area in the plane. Just getting a little hip movement during your flight may inspire someone else to do the same, and might even save them from developing a dangerous blood clot.

Blue-Blocking Glasses

This has been a complete game changer for my own travel, as there's nothing worse than being blasted by an airport's fluorescent lights after getting off a long, sleepy flight. After the sun sets, your body is hormonally setting the stage to wind down into a restorative rest mode and mend from the day's work. The blue light frequencies emitted from your cell phone, laptop, airport, bus station, grocery store, streetlight, etc., are like little artificial suns tricking your body into believing it's time to wake up. As you can imagine, this can be very hormonally confusing and spell trouble for your sleep cycles.

The issue with many of the old blue-blocking glasses is that they looked all kinds of goofy. A few options for blue-blocking glasses I recommend because they do well with both style points and protection from the artificial light are Swannies, BLUBlox, and Ra Optics. Wear your blue-blocking sunglasses at night like Corey Hart recommends in his hit song, and you'll sleep better for it.

Earplugs

Once again, these little things have saved my sanity on many a journey. You never know the potential annoying noise disruptors that could pop up once you leave the safety of your home's bedroom haven. Earplugs are certainly one of the cheapest forms of travel insurance for getting a good night's rest. I recommend grabbing the wax variety for maximum noise blocking. Ideally, you never need to use them, but for the few times you need them, you'll be immensely grateful you stashed them away. The earplugs along with an eye mask can be a powerful combination for a bit of sensory deprivation. They will also enable you to do a brief meditation in relative peace if you need to gather some energy in a tumultuous place, such as an airport.

Essential Oils for Travel

The healing and therapeutic benefits of essential oils have been enjoyed for thousands of years. There are more than 300 different essential oils available to us today. Essential oil molecules are unique in that they can actually penetrate our cell membranes and thus diffuse throughout our skin and tissues, and even get into our bloodstream.

They have the ability to move quickly throughout the body in minutes, whether applied to the skin or inhaled via the nose. Like nutrients, essential oils are metabolized by the body. However, high-quality organic and food-grade essential oils don't accumulate in the body over a period of time. The healing oils exert their action and pass on through. These natural oils can be used safely for many medicinal and health purposes. This is due to their detoxifying, stimulating, antidepressant, antibacterial, antiviral, soothing, and calming properties. They're becoming more and more widely used as a safe and cost-effective natural alternative for numerous health issues and concerns.

TOP THREE ESSENTIAL OILS TO ALIGN YOUR TRAVEL

Lavender Oil: Calm

Lavender is one of the most widely used antibacterial, antimicrobial essential oils in the modern world. When packing and preparing for your trip, it's a good idea to spray a little lavender water in and on the outside of your bags and luggage. This will prevent insects such as bedbugs and other unwelcome "guests" from hitching a ride and invading your space. Lavender water sprayed on your hotel pillows and breathed in before sleep is very calming and relaxing. You can put a few drops of the essential oil into a bath before bed to ensure a deeper, higher quality of sleep. Or mix lavender with a carrier oil to apply it directly on damp skin after bathing. This will have a softening and soothing effect on your skin, which can become dry during a flight.

Tea Tree Oil: Clean

Tea tree oil is commonly referred to as "nature's disinfectant" because it has antiseptic and antiviral properties, making it my pick for keeping you clean while traveling. It helps to provide relief from a dry scalp, dandruff, and itching associated with head lice, and helps treat eczema and dermatitis. When using tea tree oil, be sure to dilute it before applying to the skin. Diluted tea tree oil can also be used directly on the skin to control hives or to calm itching associated with eczema and dermatitis rashes. If you get the dreaded "plane cold," you can use tea tree to help treat it.

Peppermint Oil: Revive

Peppermint oil is one of the oldest European herbs; it has been used for thousands of years for its medicinal properties. For starters, peppermint can be used to soothe nausea and upset stomach. Used topically, it has a cooling effect and relieves sore muscles. Peppermint essential oil can fight infections, freshen breath, unclog sinuses, open nasal passages, and clear congestion. Studies have shown peppermint oil to be anti-inflammatory, antiviral, and to have antioxidant qualities, meaning it can help fight a respiratory infection if you pick one up while on the road.

Should you get an outbreak of seasonal allergies, especially when traveling, mix peppermint and eucalyptus oil and apply two or three drops topically to your temples, chest, neck, and back. Another perk of peppermint oil is that it can increase your energy level and improve exercise performance. Just a few deep whiffs before your movement or workout session and you will get a natural energy boost. The same goes for long road trips, studying, or anytime you need extra focus for an upcoming task.

Sitting Mechanics—Bring Spine Support

Airplane seats are designed with no consideration for optimal hip and spinal mechanics. As a responsible body operator, it's your duty to make a few subtle adjustments to save your spine while cooped up on your flight. The same way you place the bottle, pillow, jacket (or whatever you have behind your thoracic spine while driving to place your spine in a more aligned position), try that on the plane! From there, you can pull your hips all the way back to the corner of the seat to put your spine in a stacked position and fasten your seat belt to passively keep your pelvis in a healthy orientation during flight. Last but not least, I recommend using a neck pillow of some sort to maintain length in the cervical (neck) spine.

Align Band: Hotel Mobility Routine

The resistance band is light, flexible, and a minimalist's dream self-care tool for travel. It can be used as a yoga strap, exercise band, and joint mobilizer (if you have a door anchor to attach it to), and is cheaper than a gym membership. Visit TheAlignBook.com for a few simple band exercises that can be done in any hotel room while you're on the road. (We've also included a mobility routine you can do by attaching the Align Band to your car door!)

Alignment Assignment

Next time you're on the road, try this simple movement routine to assist in reversing the crummy effects of being squished in your car.

1. Six walking lunges: As you are walking away from your car, take long steps to open your hips and exaggerate them by lunging down as low as you comfortably can for six steps.
2. Clock lunges: Step out with your right foot to the twelve o'clock position for a lunge, then return back to standing, and repeat stepping with the same foot out to one o'clock. Repeat all the way to six o'clock (standing with both feet together), and then switch feet to do the same on the other side of the clock.
3. Ten jumping jacks: Stand straight with your feet together and arms by your sides. Hop both of your feet outward as you raise your arms overhead. To complete each jack, return your feet and arms to their starting positions.
4. Car-assisted shoulder stretch: Place both your hands on the side of your car as though you're being frisked. Reach your arms straight out and walk your feet away so just your hands are against the edge of the car with your thumbs facing up. Hinge your hips and bend yourself forward as in the Good Morning Stretch from Chapter 6 to stretch open your shoulders and hamstrings. Hold the stretch for thirty to ninety seconds, remembering to breathe through your nose.

CHAPTER 13

The Aligned Morning—How to Start Your Day Upright

"We are what we repeatedly do. Excellence, then, is not an act, but a habit."

—*Aristotle*

Life is far too short to allow your days to slip by without making the best of them, holding back from telling someone how much you care, or grumbling over life's minutiae. How would you start your morning if it was the most valuable day of your life? I recommend putting some real thought into that question and beginning to transfigure your morning to more closely resemble your vision. If you're interested in some ideas, here's my basic recipe for a rock-solid way to start the day.

STEP ONE: CHECK IN ON THE BREATH AND BODY

In Vipassana-style meditation, practitioners begin each day with a five-minute body scan. I've found this to be a very centering way to open the first waking moments of the day and am grateful to have learned the technique. You can practice this before going to sleep, upon waking, or anytime you'd simply like to gather your thoughts. It's super simple, too. You begin by focusing your awareness on the breath moving up through your nostrils. Once that feels easy, you can move on to exploring any varieties of sensation you experience throughout other parts of the body. You could start at the top of your head and slowly move down the side of the neck, then continue to the face, back of the neck, down the spine, etc. Once you arrive at the bottoms of your feet, work your way back up to the top of the head. Feel the sensation of pressure from the surface you're lying on, notice the contact of the sheets on your skin, and become aware of the temperature of your various body parts.

Being fully aware of sensation can be a bit tricky for the uninitiated. My personal experience with this feels like a sensation I've heard called "frisson" (the French word for shiver, referring to the sensation of goose bumps). Or you could get super fancy and call it transient paresthesia, which essentially translates to that tingling pins-and-needles sensation you may experience on the back of your neck when you watch a scary movie. With a bit of practice, you'll be able to encounter this sensation on command throughout your whole body.

Cut yourself some slack if you don't feel any sensation around certain segments or limbs at first. It takes time intentionally following the practice for your introspective awareness to become stronger. I would add that the ability to create a pins-and-needles sensation in your elbow on command is a parlor trick at best. In fact, renunciation or non-attachment to any sensation or outcome is a primary teaching in Buddhism. During Vipassana, the teacher continually reminds the students of the Sanskrit word *anitya*, meaning impermanence. Each individual sensation will certainly not last forever, so the practice of releasing attachment to "good" or "bad" feelings will come in handy for your long-term emotional well-being (which, as we learned previously, is directly associated to your physical well-being). Anything else becomes like one of those Chinese finger traps: The harder you pull away, the more the feeling cinches down upon you. Relax into the sensation, and the space is created for it to release. (This is far easier to type than actually do in practice.)

To fine-tune your sensitivity, spend a few minutes when you first wake up noticing what's going on around you and in your body. Think of your decisions first thing in the morning as setting the tone for the rest of the day. If you awake feeling stressed and rush around in a frantic effort to get out the door and to work on time, that sensation will carry over to each successive decision through the day like a stack of cascading dominoes. Try starting with a few moments of appreciation for even occupying a functional body lying on a cozy bed in the first place. Such micro-doses of gratitude and introspection might seem small, but can in fact be a high-leverage way of positioning that first domino just right to interact optimally with the next.

STEP TWO: SEA SALT, WATER, AND LEMON

The second thing I do in the morning is meander to the kitchen to grab a glass of springwater with a pinch of sea salt and a generous squeeze of organic lemon (I occasionally add a tablespoon of apple cider vinegar if I'm looking for a digestive or immune boost). Salts have been held in high regard by humanity for millennia. Even the word "salary" was derived from the Latin root word *sal*, meaning "salt." It seems logical that our deep reverence for this precious mineral for millennia is a fair indication of its health benefits.[1]

Much of the water we drink in our modern world is depleted of vital minerals called electrolytes that naturally occur when drinking directly from a spring. As the water passes through the tenuous labyrinth of rock crevices, making its arduous journey to your bottle at the surface, it's picking up a plethora of vital minerals along the way. But we modern folk have a nasty habit of sterilizing almost everything, including our water. We can get back on track by simply adding a pinch of high-quality sea salt. Pink Himalayan salt and, at the other end of the color spectrum, black Falksalt both contain more than sixty trace minerals, vital for the function of our nervous system and cell function. One of these, sodium, binds to water in the body, helping with the absorption of your morning glass of water. "But wait," I hear you say, "can't excessive salt consumption raise blood pressure?"

Well, in theory, yes. But while high blood pressure is correlated to cardiovascular disease, an analysis of eight randomized controlled trials showed insufficient evidence that the reduction of salt in one's diet prevented cardiovascular death or disease. Two further epidemiological studies on populations of 11,346 and 3,681 subjects confirmed these findings.[2] Like many things, the difference between poison and medicine is usually a question of dosage. It's time to take salt off the naughty list and re-embrace the healing mineral.

Lemons are super acidic, right? Pre-digestion, they certainly are, with a pH around two. But upon digestion, the lemons produce alkaline by-products referred to as alkaline "ash," boasting a pH above seven. It's well outside the scope of this book to explore the value of an alkaline versus acidic diet, but I will mention that the majority of the foods in the standard American diet (SAD) are more acidic. Therefore it makes sense to toss some alkaline foods into the mix when possible to balance the scales.

Lemons are also a great source of vitamin C, which we know is a strong antioxidant with huge impact on strengthening the immune system and prevention of disease (such as scurvy). In fact, one fluid ounce of lemon juice provides you with almost a quarter of your daily requirement of vitamin C. So next time you take an extended sailing trip, you know what to bring. (Limes also work— Aussies and Kiwis sometimes refer to their British brethren as "limeys" because English sailors used to suck on limes to prevent scurvy.)

In addition to their immune-boosting and pH-balancing benefits, lemons, limes, oranges, grapefruit, and other citrus fruits (we see you, tangelos) contain inflammation-reducing antioxidants that are associated with the prevention of heart disease by strengthening blood vessels and preventing the buildup of plaque, bruising, and micro-hemorrhage in the arteries, a condition of bleeding in the blood vessels.[3] It's interesting how the bitter things in life so often yield such impressive long-term benefits.

STEP THREE: INGEST THE SUN FOR BREAKFAST

"Be like the Sphinx." This is some sage advice I've received from the renowned neurosurgeon turned eccentric biohacker Dr. Jack Kruse, on a past Align

Podcast episode. The Sphinx proudly faces east, with its chest up, eyes open, feet bare. The sun has been worshipped for millennia, perhaps even giving salt a run for its money in fanfare. It represents energy, life, force, strength, power, and rebirth in a variety of religious traditions. It can purify water, give living organisms the energy needed to grow, and, of course, provide humans with a pleasant tan.

Sunlight is analogous to a musical conductor, with our hormones being the various musicians in the orchestra. That morning light sets your circadian rhythms for the day and is shown to be a key player in maintaining a consistent biological rhythm. Turns out, the Corey Hart song was spot on: Sunglasses are far healthier at night, at least since the incandescent lightbulb came to market in 1879. Our biology has been scrambling to figure out what time it is ever since.

A multitude of studies show that disruption of our daily circadian rhythm is associated with weight gain, impulsivity, slower thinking, and a host of other sub-optimal behavioral changes.[4] Our ancestors may have been on to something with their vast array of solar deities and various iterations of sun worship. Cultures around the globe spend their mornings and evenings basking in the sun's regenerating rays and tend to spend less time soaking it up when the heat of the day and UV rays are most intense, between about ten a.m. and three p.m. (depending on latitude and your ethnicity: the farther you get from the equator and the darker your skin pigment, the more midday sun you can typically tolerate and benefit from). Before and after those times, get out there if you care about your hormones.

Each morning, be sure to walk outside and expose as much of your skin as is legal and appropriate for at least a few minutes, taking solace in the fact that you're making the first step to setting up your endocrine system (and all other biological systems, for that matter) for success each day. While you're at it, grow your posture upward by raising your gaze to take in the sky, trees, and of course, sunlight.

STEP FOUR: BE GRATEFUL

This is one of the highest-leverage morning rituals I've encountered, and contrary to popular belief, you don't need to wear patch pants, paint rainbows on the side of your bus, or have a cat named Universe to contemplate the multitude of things deserving your gratitude each day.

A study done by Robert Emmons and Michael McCullough in 2003 found that counting your blessings in a daily journal increases your ability to adapt to change, reduces physical pain, and is correlated with better sleep.[5] Another study done by Rollin McCraty demonstrated that cultivating appreciation led to a 23 percent decrease in cortisol (a hormone related to stress), and 80 percent of participants experienced an increase in heart rate variability, a key indicator of health.[6] Add this happiness hack to your walk outside and ponder two or three things you're feeling gratitude for each day. Be creative with this and get specific—the dimples of a loved one when they smile or the warm feeling of sun washing over your skin.

A few more benefits of practicing gratitude include:

- Enhanced cognition
- Elevated sense of well-being
- Increased attentiveness
- Greater productivity
- Improved ability to analyze and think clearly

What is the physical weight of a single thought? I have no idea. But a positive, thankful one seems to pack a heavy punch, with a plethora of scientific evidence to back it up. My take? We need to pay closer attention to the notions that stream through our mind. It's been estimated the average person has between 60,000 and 80,000 thoughts per day, and the vast majority are the exact same as the day, week, and month before—thought habits, if you will. William James referred to living creatures as "bundles of habits"—we are pattern-based organisms, and once we lock in on a path, it can be an arduous, yet gratifying, journey to gain a semblance of control over our internal world.

Many people find writing a few thoughts of gratitude in a daily journal to be of great benefit—I recommend trying it for a week to see how it feels! Personally, I've found value in *The Five-Minute Journal* produced by my friend Alex Ikonn and co-founder UJ Ramdas. It asks what you're grateful for, what would make today excellent, and gives you a space to write out a few daily affirmations. I've also found value in having a blank notebook for what is referred to in Julia Cameron's *The Artist's Way* as "morning pages" to essentially brain-dump anything that may be rattling around in there, getting it out from between your ears and onto paper so you can move on with your life. This is a great time to get out of your phone and embrace the dying art of handwriting, which has been shown to assist with cognitive function (specifically cursive; who remembers that?!).

You may be wondering what this has to do with improving posture and movement; that's what this book is about, right? That's exactly correct, and journaling with an intention toward expression or gratitude has been shown to be helpful with relieving anxiety,[7] lowering depression scores,[8] and even reducing physical pain.[9] As we mentioned in describing the Anxious and Mopey archetypal patterns, these emotional states contort your body out of alignment. Journaling can be a safe, affordable, and restorative way to address some of the mental chatter that may be associated with chronic stress, leading to imbalanced postural patterns.

STEP FIVE: MOVE IT

Think of your body like one of those rechargeable, windup flashlights. The only way to get the bulb to shine is by winding the little handle. The human body is, of course, slightly more complex, with a myriad of handles to turn in order to spark the light, but the basic principle remains true. Each morning we wake up to an unwound flashlight, and it's not until we twist the knob that we come to life. It's so easy to understand the value in taking your dog for a walk first thing in the morning, but often it seems far-fetched to treat ourselves with the same respect.

OPTIONS TO RECHARGE YOUR "FLASHLIGHT"

- Get a kettlebell and swing it twenty times each morning.

- Take a brisk walk to some uplifting music and be willing to shake your hips, because they don't lie.

- Have your own private dance party in your living room and crank up your favorite tunes.

- Hit the gym or a yoga class.

- Go for a swim.

- Meet a buddy for a morning workout several times a week.

MOVEMENT TIP: *Hanging Leg Raises*

I like these in the morning because the technique not only opens up the shoulders (which is associated with feeling more energetic and confident, as discussed in Chapter 1) but also activates the core muscles and synchronizes your breath to movement. Get yourself a pull-up bar or find a low tree branch and let yourself hang while performing six to twelve knee-ups with legs bent or straight. Breathe in (through the nose) as your legs descend and let all your air out as you raise them as high as feels comfortable.

STEP SIX: COLD EXPOSURE

In Buddhist tradition, the root of suffering lies in desire and ignorance. We tend to desire creature comforts such as warmth, safety, and material goods, while avoiding pain and delayed gratification at all costs. Ironically, the happiest people tend to have faced a fair amount of suffering head-on. The bestselling Japanese writer Haruki Murakami is credited with saying, "Pain is inevitable, suffering is a choice." No one wants to be stuck outside in the cold, but those uncomfortable times happen to be the ones that strengthen your biology (and character) the most.

Guess what: You have a powerful tool in your home right now to practice exposing yourself to a modest micro-struggle and heroically rising up to the occasion each day. It's very simple: get into your shower and turn the handle all the way to cold. This experience literally tunes your autonomic nervous system to be less reactive to life's inevitable obstacles, translating to you being more calm, relaxed, and balanced in your body and mind. It will be uncomfortable at first, but it will eventually become a daily staple before you know it. (For the enthusiasts, you could step up your cold exposure game by grabbing a chest freezer, filling it halfway with water, and turning it on until it drops to about 50 degrees Fahrenheit for a daily plunge. For detailed instructions on how I set mine up, check out www.TheAlignBook.com.)

A British study concluded that regular cold showers increase the number of white blood cells (the disease-fighting ninjas in your bloodstream) compared to those in subjects basking in warm water. Small doses of cold can do wonders for your mental state, too. A study conducted at Virginia Commonwealth University School of Medicine found cold showers to significantly and consistently reduce feelings of depression.[10] Such benefits are connected to stimulation in the locus coeruleus in the brain, which means "blue spot" in Latin and is the center of the noradrenaline system. This area is largely responsible for our body's release of noradrenaline (also called norepinephrine), a chemical associated with combatting depression.[11] It appears our mothers, although well-meaning, were off when suggesting that cold temperatures will give you a cold. A daily cold shower can actually be a modest dose of a highly beneficial medicine.

Alignment Assignment

Try these three movements while you're out getting some morning sun:

1. **Standing Side Bend:** Start in an Aligned Standing position and raise your arms overhead while focusing on maintaining a long, neutral spine. Use your left hand to grab around your right wrist and begin side bending to the left to lengthen your whole right side. Hold this stretch for about sixty seconds and switch sides, remembering to breathe into both sides of your body.

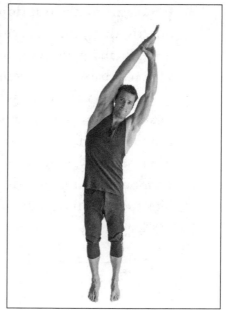

2. **Wide Leg Spinal Twist:** Start in a wide-leg stance and hinge your hips forward until your hands touch the ground (place books or a yoga block on the floor if your flexibility is limited). Maintain length in the spine and rotate to your left, raising your left hand up into the air while your right arm reaches toward the ground, creating a lengthening between your shoulders. Breathe into your thoracic spine (middle back) through your nose for three breaths and then switch sides.

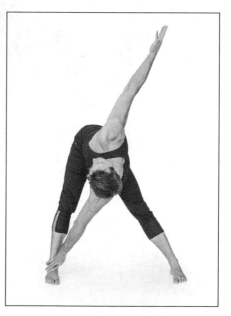

3. **Forearm Planks (Optional Hip Twist):** This is a great way to assist in activating your midsection in preparation for the day. Start on your stomach and place your forearms on the ground. Raise your torso up so you're balanced on your toes and forearms, and create a subtle lift in your abdomen (hollow position), so your low back does not sway forward. Press your shoulders forward (protraction) as though you are driving your elbows into the ground and press your toes into the ground simultaneously, so your whole body is as stiff as a board. Stay in this position for thirty seconds and remember to breathe. Try to rotate your hips to touch the ground for five repetitions on each side for an extra challenge!

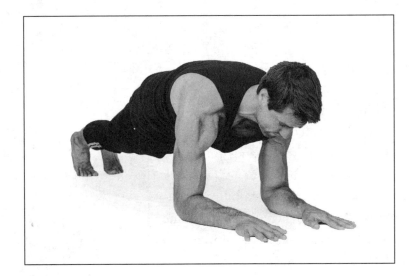

CHAPTER 14

The Aligned Evening—Accessing the Superpowers of Sleep

"A life not examined is a life not worth living."

—*Socrates*

What would you say is one of the most undervalued compounds our bodies have access to for feeling fantastic? It may be a remnant of my gym-rat background, but I'll go with anabolic steroids—the ones naturally produced inside your own body (not the scandalous variety popular among many professional athletes). One of these strength-boosting chemicals, human growth hormone (HGH), is a complex protein produced by the pituitary gland in the brain; it plays a huge role in childhood development, adult tissue quality, healthy metabolism, and may even increase life span. Big news: Experts suggest 75 percent of human growth hormone is secreted during sleep!

Want to hear a dirty little secret of the fitness industry? One doesn't really build muscle in the gym. It's that precious sleep of yours that does the work of building the body and repairing the brain. This is likely the most undervalued practice among the majority of the workaholic, hyper-productive individuals who skimp on shut-eye in an attempt to squeeze all they can from each day. They don't realize that truly "seizing the day" is only possible when you conquer the night with optimal rest. Let's begin by exploring how and where to sleep, shall we?

CHOOSING A BED

You would likely expect me to suggest you sleep on top of a straw mat thrown over a cold floor after all my heretical claims that spending more time on the ground is *actually* good for you, but you can relax. I like beds, too. Whether you're two inches from the ground on a traditional Japanese tatami mat or two feet from the ground on a traditional Western mattress, I care most about your comfort.

Technically, a lower bed will add many more squats to your lifetime, which will pay big-time dividends in hip, ankle, knee, and spine health, but you know what else is great for your joint health? Sleep, and I suggest you get as much of it as you can and truly consider your bedroom to be a restful sanctuary. I recommend investing in an organic mattress made from natural materials like wool and cotton, along with organic bedding (nobody needs to be breathing synthetic chemicals while they sleep). *What firmness should I get?* I hear you ask. According to Dr. Michael Breus, an expert in both sleep and circadian rhythms and the author of *The Power of When*, you should look for a combination of support and comfort.

SLEEP MECHANICS

A fascinating physiotherapist by the name of Michael Tetley has written extensively on the topic of sleep positions in relation to other primates, tribespeople, and the manner in which our ancestors likely spent their nights. In one article, he shows the uncanny similarities between a mountain gorilla and a Kenyan man lying on their sides to catch some ZZZ's. This is the position we will be focusing on for the sake of this book, as I am not enamored of the amount of torque placed on the neck all night via belly sleeping. or the prolonged low-back extension from sleeping on your back (for most people). That said, many sleep experts also feel that sleeping on your back can be beneficial, too. So if you're a stomach sleeper, try to start transitioning to either your side or back, using several additional pillows to pin yourself in the desired position if necessary.

At the end of the day, the most important thing is for you get to sleep—if that means you need to curl up like a bug or stand on your head to do so, I'm in support of what permits you to get ample rest. Here are some ideals I've encountered via the available research on optimal sleep mechanics for your brain and body.

WHY SIDE-SLEEPING IS ALIGNED

First of all, how do we choose a side to sleep on, and does it even matter? There is some convincing evidence that sleeping on your left side is beneficial for reducing the incidence of heartburn symptoms, which can wreak havoc on sleep. One hypothesis for why this could be is that lying on your left side keeps the junction between the stomach and esophagus above the level of gastric acid. Or it could be because right-side sleeping relaxes the lower esophageal sphincter, between the stomach and esophagus. Whatever the reason, if GERD is something you deal with at night, try sleeping on your left side and see if that helps.[1]

Circulation

Sleep specialist W. Chris Winter, MD, medical director of the Martha Jefferson Hospital Sleep Medicine Center in Charlottesville, Virginia, and author of the book *The Sleep Solution*, recommends sleeping on the left side as well for cardiovascular health. In an interview with CNN,[2] he explained that after the freshly oxygenated blood is pumped out through your body, it returns to the heart on the right side. If you sleep on your right side, you're potentially putting more pressure on the blood vessels that are attempting to carry the blood back to the heart for another pump. This should hypothetically assist in more efficient circulation (Ayurvedic medicine recommends the left side for enhanced lymphatic fluid circulation as well) and increase blood flow back to your ticker while you sleep.

Brain Health

It's also suggested by a study published in the *Journal of Neuroscience*[3] that lying on either side has brain-boosting benefits by enhancing brain glymphatic transport, which means your body more efficiently removes interstitial waste (brain gunk such as tau proteins and amyloid-beta—a peptide that accumulates in the brain of people with Alzheimer's and other degenerative brain diseases) from the brain during sleep. This study was conducted on mice, so we cannot be positive it exactly relates to humans, but better safe than forgetful.

Mechanical Pointers

All right, let's get down to business and break down some key points on how to align your sleeping position. A typical tendency is to get into a fetal position during rest. I recommend exploring what it feels like to maintain a more stacked spinal position and elongated neck, similar to if you were sitting upright on a chair but lying down instead. Here are a few key points:

- Maintain length from your sacrum to the top of your head by imagining a dowel is connected from your sacrum to the back of your head.
- Use a firm pillow high enough to keep your head in a neutral position. This involves your neck staying straight rather than too flexed or extended (which happens when your pillow is either too plump or too flat).
- Feel free to use a pillow between your arms and legs to support your shoulders and hips, but occasionally practice sleeping without them as well so as not to become dependent. At some point you may not have them, and it's wise to maintain adaptability to a variety of sleep environments.
- Remember to breathe through your nose only (refer back to Chapter 5).
- Finally, the most important thing is that you get good sleep any way you can. These are mostly ideals, and some are hypothetical at that. If your individual body may require something different—listen to what it says!

Now that we have a better sense of the mechanical components of getting a good night's sleep, let's explore a simple six-step plan to optimize your rest.

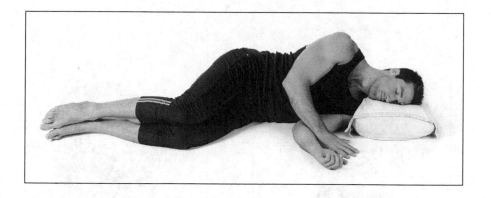

Step One: Protect Your Evening

In an old podcast episode I did with Robb Wolf, he jokingly mentioned guarding his sleep at gunpoint. It's far too easy for our personal boundaries to expand or dissipate entirely, allowing the extra work of the day to spill into the evening. Culturally, working late is far too often worn as a badge of honor, instead of a lapse of priority. You can get away with an abbreviated night's rest every now and again. Just don't make a habit of it.[4]

I challenge you to become protective of your sleep hygiene by maintaining healthy evening boundaries like setting a bedtime determined by your chronotype (think early bird or night owl with a bit more sophistication—see Michael Breus's book *The Power of When* for more on this) that you stick to more often than not and regularly granting yourself ten minutes of self-care before bed. Your new nighttime routine could include:

- Five rounds of Aligned Box-Breathing: four seconds in, hold four seconds, six seconds out, hold four seconds, repeat, sitting in an upright position and breathing through the nose only.
- Abdominal massage using fists: As you're in your sitting position from the meditation, press your fists lightly into your abdomen just above your hips creating a subtle lifting of your belly. On a breath out, lean your waist over your fists and breathe into them for approximately ninety seconds.

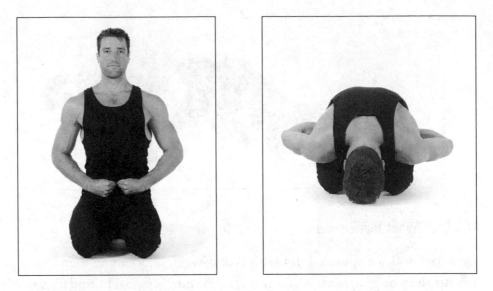

■ **Spinal Twist:** Lie on your back with your arms reaching out to the sides and slowly raise your right knee up until your right foot is on the ground a few inches from your butt. Shift your hips to the right a couple inches and then reach your right leg across your body to the left, while maintaining contact of both shoulders on the ground. If it's challenging to maintain your shoulders on the ground, try keeping the right knee bent or even bending both knees while rotating to make it a bit easier. Breathe into your thoracic spine (behind your heart) for approximately ninety seconds and then repeat on the other side.

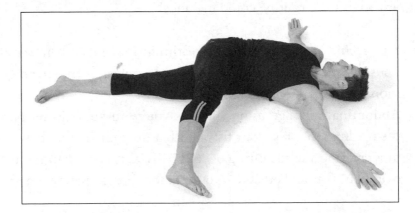

Step Two: Cut the Snacks and Late Dinners

This one is near and dear to my heart because, in the past, it has been the most challenging habit for me to break. Before I more fully understood the implications, I had the nasty habit of "eating my feelings," especially in the evening hours. The evening, after the debris of the day has settled, is often when the unaddressed emotional baggage of the week, month, or lifetime will present itself. I've heard a beautiful definition of success from an unknown source as, "being able to fall asleep when your head hits the pillow at night without feeling stress about the past or future."

For many people, this whole idea may have not resonated at all. If that's the case for you, kudos—you're winning the game of life. Regardless of why we do it, it's shown to be a biological bummer to stuff your face before bed. Researchers from Dokuz Eylul University assessed more than 700 adults with high blood pressure, examining the impact different diets and eating times had on their health.[5] They found that eating a late dinner had significant impact on overnight blood pressure. Researchers also found eating within two hours of bed produced a raised blood pressure reading, an effect even more than that of our misunderstood ally, salt. It appears your health is not just influenced by *what* you eat, but *when* you eat as well.

Another study conducted by Brazil's Universidade Federal De Sao Paulo observed the effects of late-night eating on fifty-two adult subjects ranging in age from nineteen to forty-five. This study found that evening eating consistently lowered sleep efficiency (amount of time actually asleep relative to total amount of time in bed), caused one to take longer to fall asleep, and subjects spent less time in the REM phase of sleep.[6] It gets worse! This habit then sets you up for a vicious cycle of overeating the following day, increasing the likelihood of an evening food binge due to your satiety hormones being knocked out of whack from the night of disrupted sleep.

Bottom line: What you eat matters, and so does the timing. Healthy short-term decisions build the foundation for long-term growth. Your present state of being is not a product of your last five minutes nearly as much as it is the last five weeks, months, or years aggregated together to form your present state. The body is continually keeping track of the subtle, seemingly minute decisions we make, and a key to health is consistent, long-term beneficial choices that become patterns with repetition.

If late-night eating is a habit for you, take a closer look to see if the habit is masking an undesirable sensation. Consider the possibility that stress could be addressed in more appropriate ways than a late-night burrito frenzy. I've found stepping back to do five minutes of meditation or breath work can be a beautiful way to reset when these late-night cravings come out to say "hello." Rumi said, "The cure for the pain is in the pain." Disappointingly, he never mentioned anything about the cure being found in another box of Oreos. As an alternative to nighttime snacking, try instead a gentle physical routine such as the one mentioned in the previous section to help flush out some of those feelings.

While you should avoid bingeing on junk food, a little sugar might actually help you stay asleep, as your brain uses as much glucose during REM sleep as when you're awake. If you're not diabetic or on a keto or paleo diet, then stirring a little raw, local honey in a mug of non-caffeinated tea thirty minutes before bedtime can be beneficial. If you fall into either of those categories, then skip the sweet stuff and use guava leaf tea instead.

That said, fasting and time-restricted eating (limiting food consumption to an eight-, ten-, or twelve-hour window) sometimes can also promote better sleep. A 2017 study published in *Cell Metabolism* concluded that regular fasting can reinforce healthy and consistent circadian rhythms.[7] Another paper released in the journal *Sleep & Breathing* noted that during the intermittent fasting of Ramadan, participants experienced reduced nighttime wakefulness.[8]

Step Three: Block the Blues (and Embrace Them during the Day)

Our bodies depend on healthy rhythmic cycles of all sorts, including the rhythms of light and dark in the day. One of the best ways to ensure a healthy night of sleep is to be exposed to adequate light during the day. We're like biological pendulums, and so the further we "swing" in our daytime habits, the more these will be reflected in the nighttime swing that follows.

You will experience a more robust rest side of the swing by doing your damnedest to expose your body to an adequate amount of the sun's rays during daylight hours (as discussed in Chapter 13). Get started early, as morning sun exposure prompts your body to create more of the building blocks used for melatonin, the chemical that prompts drowsiness after sundown. Remember, the rays vary depending on where the sun is relative to the horizon, and we benefit from the whole range.

Once the sun is down, or at least a couple hours before you hit the sack, start thinking about toning down the lights around your home and or using lightbulbs that don't emit the blue light frequency. This frequency of light rings your biological alarm bells, suggesting to your glands that morning has come, and it's time to get fired up! Your body releases a cocktail of stimulating stress hormones preparing you to charge forth into the rising sun, unaware that your actual intention is to sleepily watch some Netflix and hit the sack.

ALIGN YOURSELF

Some simple steps to upgrade your lighting so you can improve your sleep include:

- Get some salt lamps for rooms you frequent at night. The orange light they emit is easier on the eyes, and the salt cleanses the air.

- Check out HealthE lightbulbs, which have a light spectrum that's more conducive to restful sleep than ultra-bright LEDs.

- Grab a pair of blue-blocking glasses to wear when you don't have control of the type of evening lights, such as when you travel.

Tools and Techniques

- Download apps on your electronics to block blue light at night such as f.lux. Or just simply set your phone on the lowest light setting.

- Instate a no-screen rule in the house at least one hour before bed.

- Install an automatic timer to turn off your Wi-Fi at night and turn it back on when you need it in the morning—it's not a light thing per se, but not having the temptation to go online is a potential game changer for your sleep hygiene.

Step Four: Create Anchors

In neuro-linguistic programming (NLP) terminology, "anchoring" refers to the association of an external stimulus with an internal response. With time and repetition, it can become a powerful tool to be accessed at will. Here's what I mean: When I was eleven, I had a hockey puck signed by one of my old hockey heroes, Jaromír Jágr, from back when he played for the Pittsburgh Penguins (I grew up in Pennsylvania obsessing over ice hockey). I'd rub the puck up and down my hockey stick in a consistent pattern before every game to ensure I played a bit more like the Czech superstar.

This may sound like childish superstition, but I was actually practicing NLP well before I had ever heard the term. I was anchoring myself into a ready state by sweeping the blessed piece of rubber up and down my stick as a pregame tradition. Practices like this are no joke. It's been repeatedly shown we can augment the chemicals circulating through our bodies via environmental cues (think Pavlov's dog drooling when the bell went off signaling food time), and it's happening whether you realize it or not.

Start ingraining consistent habits of your choice around bedtime that cue you for the physiological state of rest. Bonus points if these habits are also sleep-inducing on their own, such as relaxing aromas, slow and deep massage, or a self-care routine such as the one described previously—or create one to fit your own needs. This concept is also referred to as classical conditioning, and the key, as you have probably guessed, is consistency. The cues you form become superpowers that can be called upon on demand, and once you've given them enough time to take root, they're yours for life (or as long you maintain them).

Some evening anchors I've classically conditioned myself to associate with sleep include:

- Hot cup of chamomile or reishi tea
- Journaling
- Meditation
- Putting on an eye mask
- Reading (great time for fiction) before lights-out
- My secret weapon is listening to old recordings from one of my favorite philosophers, Alan Watts. Listening to someone speak may be distracting to many people, but at this point, after many years, it's one of my most powerful tools for drifting off to sleep.

Step Five: Assess and Request

"Never go to sleep without a request to your subconscious."

—*Thomas Edison*

There is no more precious resource than your time. I repeat, there is no more precious resource than your time. Each day deserves at least a cursory glance over what went well, what you could have done better, and a setting of your intentions for the following day.

I find the structure of *The Five-Minute Journal* helpful for this, and I also derive value from scribbling my thoughts into a blank notebook; see what works for you and run with it. The key with this, as discussed in the anchors section above, is consistency. Journaling, like any habit, gains power with repetition.

This is also a potent sleep aid tool in that it gets those meandering thoughts out of your head onto paper, where they become far less disruptive upon finding a physical home. This relates to your movement and posture, because if you're stressed from thoughts constantly racing through your head or are suffering from a lack of sleep, you better believe your body shows it by holding excess tension in all those familiar sore spots!

ALIGN YOURSELF

The assess and request recipe...

- Organize your home as a part of organizing your mind.

- Give yourself the time and space for a five- to twenty-minute meditation/ self check-in.

- In your journal, write what went well, how you could have been better, and your top three intentions to make tomorrow exceptional.

- Be thankful for three things.

Step Six: Make It Black

Once you go black, you never go back. I'm referring to the level of darkness in your bedroom, of course. Did you know your skin has photoreceptors, meaning it can actually detect light? It makes a bit more common sense that an octopus or earthworm can detect light through their skin but, sure enough, humans do it, too! In recent decades, scientists have discovered extraocular photoreceptors (light-sensing cells outside of the eyes) in the central nervous system, organs, and skin! So don't think you're getting away with skimping on blackout curtains just by putting on an eye mask (although I do use one, especially for travel).[9] That said, if you, like some people, find that sleeping in pitch darkness makes it hard to wake up in the morning, then just go with the eye mask.

A dark room isn't just so you can doze off—it also affects your overall quality of sleep and is a major factor in the prevention of misaligned mental states like depression. A study published in the *American Journal of Epidemiology* found even low-level nighttime light exposure to have negative repercussions for mental health. The study measured the light emitted in the bedrooms of 863 Japanese subjects and found people exposed to more than five lux of light (ten lux is similar to looking at a candle from about a foot away) were significantly more likely to experience depression.[10] And a study published in *JAMA Internal Medicine* noted that light exposure or having a TV on in a bedroom at night caused women to gain weight.[11]

Alignment Assignment

Try these soothing movements to help wind down before bed.

1. **Happy Baby:** Lie on your back and bend your knees toward your chest. Grab the outside edges of your feet and lightly pull your feet back toward the ground. You can rock your body side to side or front to back and focus slow, deep, nasal breathing into the side of the ribs and belly. Hold this position for about ninety seconds.

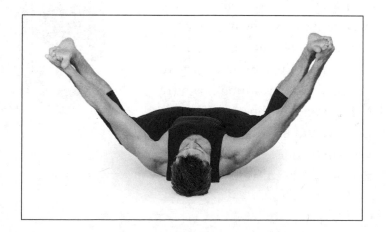

2. **Spinal Twist Shoulder Opener:** This is one of my favorite ways to open up my shoulders while mobilizing the spine. Lie flat on your belly with your arms and legs outstretched and your hands wide open and pressed into the ground. Reach your left leg over your right leg until it reconnects with the ground—this will create a lengthening through your spine and a stretching sensation in the right shoulder. Hang out in this position for about thirty to sixty seconds and then repeat on the opposite side.

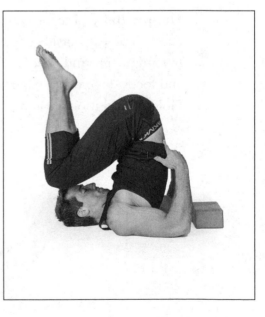

3. **Assisted Plow Pose:** Lie on your back and place a yoga block or foam roller under your sacrum, so that it lifts the sacrum and tilts it back toward your head. Bring your knees toward your chest and breathe into your belly, low back, and outside of your ribs from this position for two minutes (try to maintain nasal breathing). If you're feeling flexible, you can raise your hips off the block or foam roller and bring your knees closer to the side of your head (as shown).

PART IV

MOVING YOUR SENSES

CHAPTER 15

Near Sight—Your Eyes Need Movement, Too!

> "Looking at beauty in the world is the first step of purifying the mind."
>
> —*Amit Ray*

The typical model of fitness is one of focusing on stretching and contracting muscles as a means to alter body composition and performance. It's less common to hear of an athlete focusing on their visual acuity in a training program or a business executive harnessing the auditory spectrum for a mental edge. The truth is your senses are the foundation of your physical and mental well-being. You can leverage them as tools to discharge stress, wake yourself up, calm yourself down, or induce most any state you desire. This section will break down exactly why this is and how to begin incorporating them into your daily life for more energy, less stress, and, perhaps mostly importantly, looking better naked.

I SCREAM, YOU SCREAM, WE ALL SCREAM FOR EYE STRAIN

One of the biggest emerging health problems of our generation is the eye strain and related conditions caused by restricting vision to staring at screens that we hold right in front of us for an average of almost eleven hours each day. As frustrating as it is to have sore, red eyes, such visual restriction is also contributing to more serious conditions, including myopia (aka shortsightedness). This occurs when eyeballs keep growing beyond the point of normal development; an increasing number of optometrists and other eye health professionals are beginning to believe that the sharp spike in myopia is being caused by overuse of smartphones, iPads, and other screens.

Eye expert and co-founder of PEEK Vision Andrew Bastawrous told the UK edition of *Wired*: "People are doing more near-plane reading activity with smartphones which is encouraging the eye to become myopic to meet that environmental need. There's also evidence that suggests this is happening too quickly for it to be purely an environmental or genetic response. More recent data suggests a more important factor has been that we spend less time outdoors than we used to."[1] Not only does your depth of vision change when you're outside, taking your eye muscles through a broader range of motion, but researchers suggest regular exposure to sunlight is a crucial component to eye health as well. If you care about your vision (and posture), take off your sunglasses and move with your head held high instead of staring down into the phone when you're taking a walk outside.

While staring compulsively at screens is a major part of the vision problem that's reaching epidemic levels in some countries—in South Korea 90 percent of high schoolers are myopic—a lack of time outside is also a prime culprit. Unless you're running a daycare out of your home, indoor environments tend to be more static than outdoor ones, so there are fewer stimuli to catch your eye and cause your vision to wander as it naturally would in the wild. Indoor spaces are also far more predictable, so even their familiarity prompts less visual stimulation than when we enter a new room for the first time. Bastawrous told *Wired*, "You can walk into a room that you're familiar with and what you're actually seeing is the cached content in your internal hard drive of that room rather than actually seeing new information."

In contrast, being outdoors offers a unique visual and auditory experience every time we engage in it—provided, of course, that you're not fixated on your phone. In his bestselling book *The Rise of Superman*, Steven Kotler observes that participating in a challenging outdoor activity like skiing, downhill mountain biking, or—my favorite—surfing can quickly put you into a flow state because the novelty, unpredictability, and variability of the natural environment that you're moving quickly through is forcing your brain to focus entirely on the task at hand. This is the complete opposite of sitting on your couch for hour after hour tapping out tweets or binge-watching *Game of Thrones*. So it seems the remedy for the visual ills of being stuck indoors staring at screens is to simply allow your vision to wander outside with more regularity.

ALIGN YOURSELF

Anytime you have the chance to walk or cycle somewhere instead of driving or using public transport, take it. Use your phone calendar (irony noted) to schedule a quick outdoor break, if only for a few minutes. While you're outside, use your eyes to zoom your vision in and out from various points nearby, in the middle distance, and far away. And if you suspect you need help limiting your screen time (hey, me too!), then install an app like Freedom, Moment, or RescueTime to set better boundaries. Then use that time you're getting back to be more active, more often outside.

LOOKING UP AND OUT

"The health of the eyes seems to demand a horizon. We are never tired so long as we can see far enough."

—*Ralph Waldo Emerson*

According to the Environmental Protection Agency, American adults spend nine out of every ten waking hours indoors. This might not be quite so bad if we made an effort to frequently gaze out into nature, but while 43 percent of Americans work from home at least one day a week, many of us still spend the majority of our work time cooped up like battery hens inside office buildings.[2] And unless you happen to be a high-flying executive with a corner office or an employee at some New Agey company with a rooftop garden or indoor/outdoor space like Apple's new headquarters, you might not see the sun from the time you get to your desk in the morning until you clock out in the late afternoon (it hurts my eyes just writing it). This can be an even greater challenge during certain times of year, such as in the winter when it gets dark before quitting time.

Instead, your poor eyes face a continual, Monday to Friday, nine a.m. to five p.m. barrage of artificial light from excessively bright overhead bulbs that could be called the "junk food" of the light spectrum (you could think of it like an artificial sweetener—tastes all right but leaves you drained). This junk light from TVs, smartphones, and tablets is seeping out of those infernally bright LEDs in your office (and probably your home, too).

Dr. Alexander Wunsch, a prominent expert on photobiology, put it this way: "I call these LEDs Trojan horses because they appear so practical to us. They appear to have so many advantages. They save energy; are solid state and very robust. So we invited them into our homes. But we are not aware that they have many stealth health-robbing properties, which are harmful to your biology, harmful to your mental health, harmful to your retinal health, and also harmful to your hormonal or endocrine health."[3]

ALIGN YOURSELF

If you work in a corporate office with empty space, see if there's part of the building that offers a better view. You might not get the corner office (that'd belong to your boss—perhaps a decent enough reason to work toward becoming your own boss, just saying), but maybe you can at least score a desk with more natural light. If not, schedule as many meetings as possible in rooms with a view. And ask your boss to replace the LEDs in your office with more natural light-producing incandescent bulbs that won't damage your eyes, and if he or she won't do it, invest in some blue light–blocking glasses.

BUSTING STRESS WITH YOUR EYES

"It's not that something different is seen but that one sees differently."

—*Carl Jung*

What if I told you that you could stop chronic stress in its tracks simply by changing what you're looking at? I admit this sounds a lot like the superpower of an X-Men character (though Wolverine's claws might have a greater "wow" factor), but this isn't just the stuff of science fiction or comic books. Stanford neuroscientist Dr. Andrew Huberman's research has shown that stress and vision exist in a loop. On one end, when we experience stress, it changes our visual perception and alters the shape of our eyes. "Autonomic stress and arousal change the way you view the world around you," Huberman has been quoted as saying. "There's a physical shift that makes it easier to track a single thing, but more difficult to track multiple things in your environment."[4] This is because the sympathetic fight-or-flight state evolved to keep us alive when threatened by predators and rival tribes, so we start to home in like Chris Kyle in *American Sniper* when we perceive a threat. This may be an actual threat, like the guy who killed a mountain lion with his hands in February 2019, or an imagined one, such as traffic jams or alarmist news reports.

Fortunately, the relationship between the visual and autonomic nervous systems isn't one-way. Because it's a two-way open loop, we can use vision to modulate our stress level and reopen a panoramic view of the world. Pretty cool, right? No matter how stressed you become, you always have the power of your panoramic vision to bring you back to a calmer state.

ALIGN YOURSELF

Next time you're feeling stressed, gaze out into nature, preferably at a tree, hillside, or other green scene in the middle or far distance. In as little as forty seconds, you will start to tip the autonomic seesaw back in favor of a parasympathetic response (relax, rest, and digest). If you don't have access to such a view, looking out the window regularly will be of great help as well (open the window to allow the full spectrum of light to enter the room). Finally, get a photo or two printed of mountains or the beach to put on your walls for an extra dose of nature therapy. That's better for your eyes (and mental state) than staring at the same picture on a screen.

TUNNEL VISION

If an angry-looking lion ran into the room, you'd have some obvious physical reactions, like leaping to your feet, trying to find the nearest exit, grasping for a makeshift weapon, and perhaps even dropping this book. (Don't worry, I'm not offended—surviving an attack by an apex predator comes before finishing this chapter.) But there'd also be some less obvious reactions. One is your peripheral vision shrinking, and your peepers concentrating on only what's in front of you—in other words, tunnel vision. Your survival now depends on you being aware of the lion's every move and mobilizing each muscle, sinew, and iota of energy to either kill it, escape, or die trying. And this all-out effort is in part conducted by focusing your eyes on the 500-pound ball of muscle that wants to tear you limb from limb.

Maybe that's a silly, overly dramatic scenario. But even lesser stressors create changes in your visual system similar to outrunning an oncoming, growling prehistoric death-machine. When we're in a busy, frenetic environment like a bustling city street, the New York subway, or the London Underground, we're in a state of continual vigilance, ready to respond to the potential threat posed by fast-moving traffic, loud noises (see Chapter 16), and running late for that important meeting. In a paper published in the *International Journal of Environmental Research and Public Health*, researchers found looking at photos of cities after being exposed to a stressor either made participants feel more anxious or didn't improve their recovery from the stimulus. In contrast, those who were shown pictures of nature reduced their anxiety. The difference? The cityscape triggered the sympathetic nervous system (be on your guard!), while the photos of a forest prompted a parasympathetic response (relax).[5]

On top of our eyes continually reacting to the environment, our actions and behaviors can prompt alterations in our vision which are inextricably tied to the state of the autonomic nervous system. One of these is staring at a screen for hours on end. By doing so, we're voluntarily reducing the entire world to a tiny field of vision that extends no more than a few inches in front of our faces. On one level, electronic device addiction is creating physical changes in our eyes. One study found a large quantity of screen time narrows the blood vessels in children's eyes, which is an indicative marker of early-onset cardiovascular disease. In contrast, kids who spent more time being active outdoors without a cell phone or tablet had healthy retinal vasculature.[6]

Most of us cannot completely avoid looking at screens, or even want to. But you don't have to become a tech teetotaler to improve how you treat your eyes and, in turn, enhance your autonomic nervous system tone (like toning your six-pack, but more important). First, try taking a break from the news cycle or at least limit your exposure to checking the headlines just once a day. Then, start batching your email and social media use into specific times of the day instead of it being open season all year long.

ALIGN YOURSELF

When you have to be in front of your computer for an extended amount of time, set a timer for twenty-five minutes. Each time it goes off, get up (from the floor hopefully) for a much-needed eye break by taking a five-minute stroll while staring at various distances, including the horizon. Feel free to throw in some lunges, squats, or jumping jacks for an extra movement boost.

LET THERE BE DARK

"The only thing worse than being blind is having sight but no vision."
—*Helen Keller*

In the Czech Republic, there's a term you won't find in any guidebook: *terapie tmou*. While this sounds like some sort of tasty chocolate dessert—or maybe I'm just hungry—the phrase actually means "darkness therapy." That's right—healing yourself with an absence of artificial light. The good people at the Beskid Rehabilitation Center and many other Czech wellness retreats believe that spending up to a week in total darkness can alleviate a wide variety of issues, including sleep disturbances, depression, and social jet lag (when your body clock and lifestyle get out of synch). Marek Malůš, a professor of psychology at the University of Ostrava's Faculty of Arts, says that darkness therapy is a form of REST, restricted environmental stimulation therapy—a ritzy name for sensory deprivation.[7] His research has found that people who participate in a week of dark therapy experience a significant reduction in anxiety and feelings of depression.

A form of this technique that is more popular in the West is isolation tanks, which combine light restriction with hydrotherapy. Everyone from psychonauts like Joe Rogan to pro sports studs such as two-time NBA MVP Steph Curry or biohackers like Ben Greenfield rave about the relaxation-promoting benefits of closing off the outside world, turning off the lights, and floating in mineral-rich water that mimics the elevating effects of the Dead Sea. But rather than having to fly to the Middle East, you can likely find a few flotation/isolation pods at your local spa. And the results aren't merely anecdotal—a paper published in the peer-reviewed journal *BMC Complementary and Alternative Medicine* concluded that "Stress, depression, anxiety, and pain were significantly decreased whereas optimism and sleep quality significantly increased for the flotation-REST group."[8]

You don't have to fly to the Czech Republic and spend a week in darkness or push your claustrophobic boundaries in an isolation tank to reap some of the benefits. A more affordable option is to find a peaceful area in your home as a space to retreat. Simply lie down in a darkened room (draw the curtains, remove all electronics, cover any light sources), throw on an eye mask if any light is creeping in, close your eyes, and listen to relaxing music for twenty to forty minutes (silence is a great option too). This would be a fantastic opportunity to practice a breathing technique (see Chapter 5, on nose breathing) or simply be with yourself for some quiet introspection (see Chapter 18, on mindfulness).

FOCUS ON YOUR FEET

How do you avoid tripping over the stray bucket that a building crew kindly left on the sidewalk, dodge passersby in a busy airport, or even avoid falling over your own feet? Adaptive locomotion. Your eyes are constantly monitoring your surroundings and making micro-adjustments to your balance and positioning in three-dimensional space. Most are imperceptible, except when you need to leap away from that lunging Rottweiler or leap back from the crosswalk when that Hummer you were sure was going to stop doesn't. Your visual, vestibular, and musculoskeletal systems are in a state of constant interplay, like the various sections of a well-conducted orchestra.

Unless, of course, you're gazing down at your phone like a zombie. We've all had to step aside to let someone blunder by with absolutely no awareness of what's going on around them because Instagram apparently cannot wait. Sometimes I envision "Terrible" Terry Tate flying out of nowhere to go all "Office Linebacker" on this distracted person. But the clueless phone addict isn't just compromising their own short-term safety or annoying the bejesus out of the rest of us—they might actually be hindering their ability to effectively move through the world. Researchers at the University of Columbia found that people who text during perambulation (walking) move more slowly and are, perhaps unsurprisingly, unsteady on their feet.[9] Worse still, a study published in *Frontiers of Psychology* states that loss of anticipatory control and the resulting change in adaptive locomotion can increase fall risk in the elderly and start to mirror the destabilizing effect of Parkinson's disease.[10] Remember, you're always training your movement (and thought) patterns—each step is a practice and opportunity to become more balanced or, in the case of the cell phone, more distracted and unstable.

The remedy isn't complicated. Focus on your footfalls, not your phone, and try to look up, down, out, and around you instead of just seeing what's right in front of your face. If you watch your kids, grandkids, nieces, or nephews when they're outside, you'll probably notice that their head and neck act like a gyroscope—always twisting, turning, and tilting to look at something new and exciting. Contrast this to how most of us adults walk around with our gaze fixed firmly in front of us or looking down at our precious phones.

As we get older, we seem to lose our sense of wonder at the world. Re-expand your sense of wonder by simply extending your scope of vision. According to Florence Williams, *Outside* magazine contributor and author of *The Nature Fix*, "We'll get the biggest bang [for our nature-immersing/vision-restoring buck] when we turn off the devices" and "listen to birds, watch clouds and the sunset."[11]

ALIGN YOURSELF

Take a walk, and put your phone into Do Not Disturb mode so only your nearest and dearest can contact you in an emergency (I personally choose airplane mode, but to each his or her own). Focus on what's going on around you—just because you can do two things at once doesn't mean it's the best decision. This is particularly true when you're on a trail or walking alongside a body of water. If you want to get all the stress-busting benefits nature can provide, remain fully engaged by putting your tech toys away.

Consider shedding your shoes because the high density of nerves in your feet can further increase your proprioception and, as Richard Louv writes in his book *Vitamin N*, "Barefoot walkers are more likely to look down, to take care of where they step and are less likely to fall. Walking barefoot enhances awareness of texture and terrain."[12]

EYE EXERCISE ROUTINE AND ITS BENEFITS

We've talked a lot of theory in this chapter. Now it's time to leave you with some practical takeaways. We enlisted the help of my good friend Ryan Glatt, brain health coach and psychometrist at Pacific Brain Health Center, for his go-to eye exercises to improve brain health. Performing them every day will not only help your vision, but will also have a beneficial knock-on effect for your physical health, mental acuity, and emotional well-being. Before we get to the exercises themselves, let's first examine why they're helpful.

Biomechanics

Due to being fixated on our screens—laptop, phone, TV, or otherwise—for hours every day, we are typically in a posture that is sub-optimal and often asymmetrical. For example, many individuals look at the phone near where they removed it from their pocket; down and to the right. This rotates the rib cage and the head toward that same vector, and causes a "battle" with the muscles on the opposite side of the body. Some may become lengthened, others may become shortened. The point is, you are causing a musculoskeletal argument, when everyone was getting along just fine without your compulsive lower-diagonal phone-checking. (By the way, it doesn't look any cooler to glance down at your phone that way.)

This can lead to torsions (not permanently, but there is potentially the development of a neuromuscular bias) in certain parts of the body that may manifest as tightness in weird places, such as one side of the back of your skull, the side of your neck, a strange part of your lower back that you can't seem to place, etc. This same disruption also occurs when you hold a coffee cup or phone while walking, which can disrupt the important "contralateral swing" of the arms that is so important to healthy gait (see the *Seinfeld* episode in which Elaine's colleague doesn't swing her arms when she walks, and so lurches about like a cave dweller). So whether it's a static posture or a dynamic motion, ipsilateral-visual-fixations may compound over time to be sensationally annoying, and even potentially increase injury risk or cause pain.

Nervous System

As discussed previously in the chapter, our autonomic nervous systems can be affected by our vision. For example, we are often stuck in central "fixed" vision; focused on a single target in front of us, often positioned or near-positioned centrally. Spending too much time in central vision can not only cause fatigue, but possibly increase the tone of the sympathetic nervous system, triggering the fight-flight-freeze mechanism and all the neurochemical and psychological goodies that can come with it. These include persistent anxiety, chronically elevated cortisol that leads to disease-breeding inflammation, and sleep disruption.

On the other hand, panoramic vision—the more "expansive" field of view—may have the opposite effect, leading to an engagement of the parasympathetic system, helping us to potentially achieve the ever-valuable rest-and-digest response that so many of us suppress with our always-on lifestyles. This is probably why looking out at a beautiful, expansive view in nature may deliver the deep sigh of relief, wonder, and relaxation that so many of us crave—maybe we are just too centrally bound all the time via our vision.

Some simple potential applications include:

- Not staring at your phone while eating; that is central vision and may trigger sympathetic response, which is not helpful for digestion.

- Not staring at your phone while pooping (I love this one), because it does the opposite of rest-and-digest due to centralized binding. Space out while you poop with a view instead.
- Get outside not just for the exercise, but for the change in vista.
- People who look "spaced out" seem to look like their eyes are stuck on a panorama. If you start feeling spacey, focus on something central without distractions.
- People who are hyper-focused or super stressed probably need to space out more. Stare into space or look at a horizon for a few minutes and see how you feel.
- Anxious people seem to have their eyes dart around the room a lot. Perhaps fixating on something soothing or enjoying the sensation of panorama could help.

GENERAL VISUAL HEALTH

As we age, we gradually lose what is called "the general visual field of view," which leads to visuospatial deficits, loss of functional and independent activities, and even getting your driver's license revoked because of poor vision and insufficient perceptual-cognitive abilities to react to the dynamic, ever-changing environment that is the road. In addition, the most common neurodegenerative disease is macular degeneration, affecting many times more people than dementia. While people may have various viewpoints on the topic (most agree that a healthy lifestyle prevents these age-related visual deficits), giving your eyes some variable movement and keeping them "fresh" cannot hurt! Here are six simple exercises to strengthen and mobilize your eye muscles; you can think of it as yoga for eyeballs!

1. Horizontal Saccades

Keeping your head still while sitting or standing, stick your arm straight out in front of you, as if you're giving an enthusiastic thumbs-up. Start moving your arm (and therefore your thumb) across your body horizontally left and right, back and forth. You can think of a metronome going side to side at a steady rhythm. Let your eyes follow the tip of your thumb, which will result in a steady left-to-right eye movement, almost as if you were scanning the horizon. Do not let your eyes leave the tip of your thumb, as staying focused on it and not being distracted by external factors is important. As you move your arm back and forth, extend it out all the way each time until your hand is as far away from your face as possible. Repeat this and the following exercises for one minute. If during any of these exercises, you feel any eye strain, headache, dizziness, nausea, or fatigue, you can reduce the speed, distance, or duration of the exercise.

2. Vertical Saccades

Keeping your head still while sitting or standing, stick your arm straight out in front of you, as if you're giving an enthusiastic thumbs-up. Start moving your arm (and therefore your thumb) vertically, up and down your body. Let your eyes follow the tip of your thumb, which will result in a steady eye movement up and down, almost like looking toward the sky, then toward the ground, without moving your head.

3. "X" Saccades

Keeping your head still while sitting or standing, stick your arm straight out in front of you, as if you're giving an enthusiastic thumbs-up. Start moving your arm (and therefore your thumb) in a diagonal direction, similar to making a big "X" across your body. Let your eyes follow the tip of your thumb, which will result in a steady eye movement diagonally, almost like looking in the upper corner of a room and then down toward the ground outside of your opposite hip, without moving your head.

4. Near-Far Switches

Keeping your head still while sitting or standing, stick your arm straight out in front of you, as if you're giving an enthusiastic thumbs-up. Then, choose a target in the distance (a spot on the wall, a distant tree outside, a street sign, the handle of a door down the hallway, etc.), ideally several feet away. Look at the thumb close to you, and then look at the chosen target (precisely!) that is farther away. Keep switching between the two targets, as we're typically used to focusing centrally on a target in front of us.

5. Panoramic-Central Switches

Keeping your head still while sitting or standing, stick your arm straight out in front of you, as if you're giving an enthusiastic thumbs-up. Then, choose a landscape in the distance or on the horizon (a parallel street, a mountain, a distant freeway, etc.), ideally as far away as possible. If you have ever been seen a lovely view and taken a deep breath or sighed while appreciating its beauty, that is the mechanism we are trying to replicate here. Look at the thumb close to you, and then look at the panoramic landscape. Keep switching between the two viewpoints; central and panoramic. If you feel like it, stare at the panoramic view for longer.

If you cannot find a sound panoramic view (such as when you are indoors), pretend! Imagine looking out from a beautiful mountain range, staring out to sea (like you're in Malibu), or focusing your gaze on a forest (like in Yosemite Valley), or whatever else strikes your fancy. Of course, you want to conjure this sensation without closing your eyes, and the feeling might include "spacing out," or feeling like your eyes are moving away from your nose. Try not to get distracted by other moving targets in either field of view. Repeat this for one minute. Remember, if you feel any eye strain, headache, dizziness, nausea, or fatigue, you can reduce the speed, distance, or duration of this exercise.

6. Wall Ballers

Get a tennis ball and stand about three to four feet away from a wall. Hold the ball at shoulder height, and initiate a gentle overhand (or underhand if it's easier) toss against the wall, ideally at a height a few inches above your head. Catch the ball, being sure to grasp it in a quick, strong fashion as it comes back to you. The motion of the ball should be a smooth arc, equaling a quarter of a miniature rainbow. Repeat this faster if you are up for it, and let your eyes follow the ball for an extra visual workout. Get closer if you're feeling dangerous, and do not be discouraged as you get used to the exercise. Perform fifty repetitions on each side.

For extra fun, replace the wall with a person and play a dynamic, short-lived, visual-health-focused session of catch. For extra challenge, get two tennis balls and throw and catch them with both hands at the same time, or throw and catch them in an alternating fashion (wall ball juggling?). Some fighters and boxers get farther away from the wall and even do "wall ball boxing," where they juggle the ball up in the air against the wall using only their fist (hard but super rewarding). If you want to do this but just can't get the hang of doing it with a ball, use a balloon to get some extra hang time.

Alignment Assignment

Start paying more attention to the ceiling of every room you walk into as a way to raise your gaze, open your posture, and de-stress your mind. Make a point to look out into the horizon regularly each day and sprinkle in some gratitude as you do so for good measure.

Try one of the eye exercises mentioned above each day this week until you've successfully done them all. If one feels more challenging than the others, put more focus on that technique until it becomes easy. If you'd like to try the expert version of the exercises, remember to smile while you're practicing.

CHAPTER 16

Finding Your Voice—the Way Sound Moves Us

"Without music, life would be a mistake."

—*Friedrich Nietzsche*

For years, neuroscientists believed that music was processed the same way as any other kind of sound. But recent research cited by Steve Connor in *The Independent* demonstrates that there's a specific group of neurons in the auditory cortex that are only activated by listening to music, meaning we can distinguish on a cellular level between it and other, non-musical sounds such as speech (which the study authors also connected to a distinct group of neurons).[1] This suggests there may be other responses to music in the body and brain that we have not yet discovered.

Of course, music isn't *merely* a neurological thing. Has a song ever reduced you to a crying, quivering mess? Or have you been at a show with friends and felt an overwhelming sense of rapture that seems to not only wash over you but entrain the entire crowd into one swaying organism? The affective power of rhythmic sound is one of the reasons it's universal and present in literally every culture across the globe, regardless of geographic location, economic status, race, etc.

Music is a life force permeating literally every society. It's as crucial a part of any cultural motif as food, and the best part—it's also an anti-fragile, renewable resource that only gets more profound under stress. Rhythmic sound has been a facilitator for the optimal functioning of human biology in shamanistic cultures for thousands of years. Archaeologists have found instruments dating back as far as 43,000 years, such as the Divje Babe flute made from the femur of a cave bear found in Slovenia. Think about that: Your ancestors were holed up in caves more than 40,000 years ago while avoiding being prey and still felt an innate urge to carve a wild animal's leg bone into a sound maker for their own wellness.

Music is the perfect translation for the human experience, free of the constraints and potential deception entwined within spoken language. When a person feels understood at the deep, visceral level that only the undefined languages of touch, dance, and music can access, the physical body and psyche begin to relax, granting permission to be taken on a journey of feeling instead of the necessity to always drive the train.

We also have the non-musical sounds like the soothing burble of a mountain stream or the cacophony of police sirens, honking cars, and construction equipment in a city. The sonic component of every environment has an impact on our nervous system, mood, and, like music, even our cellular biology. In this chapter, we'll compare and contrast different aural environments, and also give you some ways to fine-tune your home and headspace so you can benefit from calming sounds while recovering from overexposure to the harsh ones.

A WORD ABOUT QUIET

On the other end of the sound spectrum lies silence. Amidst the clamor and bustle of our modern lives, we rarely encounter true quiet accidentally, and most of us do little to purposefully create even a few seconds of unadulterated silence in our daily lives. Yet being still and quiet is a powerful discipline that can help us mentally reset, physically chill out, and manipulate our mood so we become stronger human beings. Have you ever been deep in the wilderness, miles away from any semblance of human contact, and noticed an almost eerie quietness? It's as though you're on another planet. The vast emptiness can feel uncomfortable and even a bit creepy to a person unaccustomed to basking in a moment void of distraction.

As a society, we've tuned out silence for so long, it feels uncomfortable being alone with our thoughts for even a brief interlude. Yet carving out a little time for silence and solitude can have a profound impact on our emotional, physical, and spiritual well-being. In the next few hundred words, I'll show why music, sound, and silence matter more than you likely thought, and how to utilize them going forward to enrich your life.

HEALING SOUNDS

A study of 6,000 adult Americans found that 51 percent of women and 60 percent of men had suffered at least one life-altering traumatic event in their lifetime, with 8 percent struggling with chronic post-traumatic stress disorder (PTSD).[2] Over the past decade, we've started to see alternative treatments to medication gaining traction in both military and civilian populations. One of the most popular and effective is musical intervention. Though there have been only four major clinical studies to empirically investigate the clinical impact of sound, they all suggested that music helps PTSD sufferers avoid fixating on recollections of their traumatic experiences, reduces perceived stress and anxiety, boosts self-confidence, and lowers levels of the stress hormone cortisol. Group-based music therapy was also shown to improve social connections, which creates further calm through an increased sense of belonging to a caring community.[3]

So how exactly does all this work at the neurological level? One of the mechanisms is believed to be the way that music calms down the amygdala, the part of the brain responsible for modulating fear and anger. This area can become hyper-sensitized during repeated exposure to high-stress events, such as soldiers who are in firefights day after day for an entire tour of duty, or a lawyer who works eighty-hour weeks. Rhythmic sound seems to reset the amygdala back to a more normal baseline by taking it out of a high-alert state.[4]

It has also been proven that listening to and performing music increases blood flow to the ventral striatum, orbitofrontal cortex, and other areas of the brain involved in regulating emotion and reward-based responses. Simultaneously, both the creation and consumption of sound triggers a release of dopamine, endorphins, serotonin, and other pleasure-related hormones, which can help replace sadness with joy.[5] A meta-analysis even found listening to music and playing an instrument can trigger neurogenesis, which is a fancy term for the creation of new brain cells.[6]

ALIGN YOURSELF

If you're feeling stressed out or overwhelmed, purposefully set aside some time to play your instrument of choice (this includes the oldest human instrument, your voice box). Or stack some tension-relieving techniques such as walking outside in the fresh air under the sun with some of your favorite music in your earbuds. Your body enjoys stacking wellness variables; take advantage of that and bring your music outside. Perhaps take your shoes off, and maybe you could even go nuts and pass a smile to another human (sounds a lot like a music festival; no wonder they're so popular).

YOUR EMOTIONAL REMOTE CONTROL

"Did you know that our soul is composed of harmony?"

—Leonardo da Vinci

Singing transforms a passive experience—listening to music—into an active, participatory one, literally making you part of the song. It can help you empathize more with the feeling the singer is conveying, or you might come up with your own emotional take on a song. Sometimes we sing to lift ourselves up, as in a scene from *Night at the Roxbury*, and at other times we're feeling more contemplative and an Amy Winehouse–style melody is better to navigate through the introspective terrain.

The various tones produced in song are like keys for unlocking specific states of mind. Here's an interesting excerpt from *The Polyvagal Theory in Therapy* by Deb Dana on the way sound conducts the state of your nervous system:

> Through a Polyvagal perspective we know the autonomic nervous system responds to sound. Certain frequencies activate ventral vagal safety and others signal danger and a move into sympathetic or dorsal vagal survival responses. Low frequency sounds bring a neuroception of danger with an autonomic reminder of long ago predators. Your client's focus shifts from social connection to survival actions. High frequency sounds take your clients out of connection into concern as their attention shifts to the source of the sound. Unpredictable sounds from outside the therapy office door can activate protective reactions.[7]

This paragraph is geared toward therapists but relates to all human interaction. You can look at the power of sound as an emotional remote control and your present state as the image projected on the screen. Here's how the controller works: Choose your desired state, find music that matches said state, belt it out (dance along with it, if you prefer the image to be in HD), and witness your internal channel change.

Listening to what Dr. Stephen Porges refers to as a prosodic voice (one with pleasing tone and rhythm) is certainly good for you, but you also want to engage your own voice prosody to get all the soothing sonic benefits! By activating the muscles in the back of your throat, singing stimulates the vagus nerve, which triggers a relaxation response via the parasympathetic (rest-digest) nervous system. And that blissful feeling you sometimes get when you're sing-ing like nobody's watching? It comes from the release of the pleasure hormone oxytocin, which bursting into song like a morning lark triggers.[8]

MECHANICS OF SINGING AND SPEAKING

Remember in Chapter 1 when we discussed that your posture is connected to how you feel? Well, it's also foundational for how you sing and speak! Your body is an instrument of expression, and the richness of the tones projected is a product of the shape and tune of the instrument (your postural patterns).

Your voice can project you to be strong, confident, and stable, or weak, unsure, and out of control based on the tone, rhythm, pitch, and pacing of your language. As we've learned, it doesn't just affect the way other people feel about you—you're literally tuning your own nervous system as you speak (or sing)! When your body is in alignment, your vocal cords are set up to project across a large room or speak with confidence in an intimate space.

There's good news: You don't need to learn a special singing posture, because the Aligned Standing principles we discussed in Chapter 6 are consistent with what you'd learn from a singing coach. In case you haven't noticed the pattern, the fundamental principles of moving well discussed in Part II are consistent with most any modality of movement, including speech and song!

Here are a few postural pointers to help align your voice:

- Feet about shoulder-width apart
- Slight micro-bend in knees
- Neutral pelvis (Try squeezing your butt muscles and notice what happens to your pelvic orientation: This will be closer to neutral. Then try to relax your butt while maintaining the position.)
- Level your ribs to be stacked over your pelvis to avoid the ribs flaring upward.
- Relax the shoulders and hands. (Think of your hands as tools to guide your vocal expression, like a musical conductor manipulating a baton to guide an orchestra.)

■ Imagine a string is slightly pulling the back of your head upward toward the sky to lengthen your spine.

I learned this exercise from my friend, the Broadway star Carrie Manolakos, during a singing lesson recently. In order to train breath capacity to hold longer notes (which she does like no one else I've heard), she recommended this technique: Start in the Aligned Standing position and place your hands on the sides of your ribs. Take your largest nose breath in by expanding your ribs out to the sides, and as slowly as you can, begin breathing out all of your air, making a *shh* sound with your mouth. You can also do this same technique while slowly rolling your spine down into a forward fold and repeating on the way back up to standing.

KEEP HUMMING ALONG

Certain kinds of meditation involving humming and chanting can also trigger positive physical and emotional effects, due to the resonance of the vibrations created. One Indian brain imaging study found using the "om" chant during yoga quiets the region of the brain associated with depression.[9] Another yoga humming technique called Bhramari involves buzzing like a bee. A paper published in the *Journal of Traditional and Complementary Medicine* found this time of pranayama reduces blood pressure, encourages parasympathetic recovery, and reduces stress.[10]

The same paper noted people who hummed reported feeling blissful and said their mind felt refreshed afterward. This is in large part because humming on the exhale lengthens the overall duration of each breath and reduces the number of breaths per minute; it helps to rebalance the autonomic nervous system and encourage a transition from feeling stressed out to relaxed.[11] To tap into these benefits, simply breathe in through your nose and then hum as you breathe out through you nose.

TECHNIQUE

Bhramari Pranayama

A brief disclaimer: This one looks a little weird—OK, it looks very weird—but it works wonders to calm your nervous system and create a little mental reset. It's reminiscent of what a child may naturally do when they feel overwhelmed and need to calm down (it's interesting how often the natural self-care practices of kids and animals will look a lot like what adults pay big money to learn). It's really simple to do. Start by using your thumbs to close your ears by lightly pressing the cartilage of your ear over the ear canal. Then with both ears plugged, close your eyes and take a full breath in through your nose and make an *mmmm* sound for as long as you have air to make it happen. Repeat this six times and check in with how you feel.

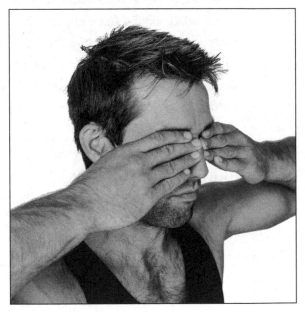

Piping Up to Wind Down

Have you ever wondered why they do that long-winded "om" at the beginning and end of some yoga classes? Yes, it's said to represent the original sound of the universe. That's cool, but who the heck really knows what the initial sound of creation was like in the first place, and how does that help me pay my bills or finally get me into a handstand?

More tangibly for your day-to-day use, you're activating those same restorative parasympathetic switches in your body via emphasizing a long out-breath while exhaling any stagnant bits of air in your lungs. The sound is actually pronounced A-U-M, with the M part being a closed-mouth *mmmm* sound, followed by silence. Yes, each of the distinct syllables (including the silence afterward) have deep symbolic meanings, but for the sake of this book, let's stick to its physiological effects. The creation of each sound causes the reverberation to be focused on a different part of your head and thorax like a biologically built-in sonic massage system. Not to mention, the effects of this tradition along with other forms of breath practice (pranayama, if you prefer yoga speak) have been scientifically shown to improve pulmonary function, increase mental alertness, relieve stress, and even resolve depression via stimulation of the vagus nerve![12]

ALIGN YOURSELF

Next time your significant other drags you to a yoga class, you can appreciate the science-based benefits of the long and at times perhaps slightly awkward group humming experience that may ensue. Start integrating the same principles while you're driving or any time you're feeling a little stressed: Simply belt out a few long-winded hums or oms, and feel free to explore a variety of pitches while doing so, then check back with how you're feeling.

MUSIC AND MEMORY

Ever heard couples claiming, "This is our song," when a certain tune starts piping in through your local coffee shop's speakers? Of course you have. And you've likely got several songs that you'd claim as your own, too. Each one is probably tied to a different time, place, and/or person. We can link music in our minds to positive periods in our lives—like going to a summer festival with your high school besties (the kind of fond remembrance that psychologists call a "reminiscence bump")—or sad ones, such as a relationship breakup or the passing of a loved one. Consciously, we comprehend that songs are tied to emotions, locations, seasons of life, and so on. Yet in the subconscious mind, the associations run much deeper, like a subterranean river.

Rather than just involving one part of your noggin, listening to and performing music fires up extensive neural networks and lights up huge swathes of the brain like one of those satellite photos showing the twinkling lights of big cities against the blackened expanse of the night sky. When we have a recollection prompted by hearing a familiar oldie, fMRI scans show that the prefrontal cortex bursts into life. The more vivid the memory, the more activity is sparked in this part of the brain. In an article for *Psychology Today*, Daniel Bergland explained that listening to music also triggers a potent response in areas tied to creativity, cognitive processing, and even movement.[13] The latter hints at why music and dance go together so naturally— they're literally hardwired together in a dynamic neural circuit in our brains.

Collective singing can be just as potent. Harmonizing in a group, whether in a choir, at a concert, or during a road trip with your buddies à la Harry and Lloyd in *Dumb and Dumber*, has been found to increase heart rate variability (HRV)—more variability is better, because it indicates fuller recovery from stressors and a greater balance in the autonomic nervous system than low variability. Interestingly, it wasn't just the singers' voices that synchronized, but also their heart rates and HRV.[14] Group singing is also good for your mood. A six-month study in England discovered that those who participated in a weekly singing group improved their overall mental health and reported feeling more positive and able to cope with their problems.[15]

One of my favorite slightly outlandish activities is the Monday Night Kirtan here in Santa Monica, where folks spend the evening doing call-and-response singing along with dancing. After a couple hours it feels a whole lot like the purgative effects of many spiritual practices, just sweatier. Song seems to supersede religious dogma and strike a chord deeper than intellectual thought—it's like a nameless, faceless, deep web connecting all of humanity. Our only responsibility is to trust it and dive in.

Find five songs you love that make you feel energized, and make a playlist. (You can even call it your Align Playlist!) Listen to it in the mornings or when you're doing some of the other movements in the book. Change it and update it with new music as new songs strike your fancy, but starting a positive association between the moves in this book and your musical experience will help you stick to the habit and feel great doing it. And, per that same *Psychology Today* article, be sure to dance if you want an even richer musical experience.

SO YOU THINK YOU CAN DANCE?

"Dance is the hidden language of the soul."

—*Martha Graham*

There's a reason that, like music, dance is universal: It's a way to nonverbally communicate powerful emotions, demonstrate cultural flair (think of those debonair Brits with their Lambeth walk or fiery Latinos and the flamenco), and let loose. A twenty-one-year study conducted by the Albert Einstein College of Medicine in New York discovered that while reading reduced the chance of developing dementia by 30 percent and doing crosswords and similar puzzles by 47 percent, dancing was the most effective preventive measure, reducing the incidence of dementia by a whopping 76 percent.[16]

In a commentary on the study, Stanford University dance instructor Richard

Powers explained the reason for this brain-protecting power of the polka, waltz, and any other style: "Dancing integrates several brain functions at once—kinesthetic, rational, musical, and emotional—further increasing your neural connectivity."[17]

Another paper published in the *British Journal of Sports Medicine* concluded that while physical exercise and a free-form dance class both improved mood by around 25 percent, the latter had a greater impact on participants' creativity. The authors suggest, "The slightly greater improvements in creativity after aerobic dance could possibly be due to the nature of the exercise, which allows more freedom of movement than the regimented aerobic workout."[18] So while there's nothing wrong with a structured workout, you might also do well to cut loose more often and dance like nobody's watching.

ALIGN YOURSELF

You don't have to become Fred Astaire or Shakira to reap the brain- and body-boosting benefits of dance. My experience is that dance classes are very open and welcoming to all levels and body types of movers. Try starting with a partner dance like bachata or tango for the social engagement or Zumba, West African, dance hall, break dancing, or hip-hop for a more physically demanding experience.

THE SOUND OF SILENCE

Every faith tradition refers to and encourages the combination of silence and solitude. In the Bible, we are told, "Jesus went out to a mountainside to pray, and spent the night praying to God. When morning came, he called his disciples to him." (Luke 6:12–13) Buddhist texts also contain frequent references to silence and solitude, with the Buddha saying in the Sutta Nipata, "One should wander solitary as a rhinoceros horn."[19] Elsewhere in Buddhist literature, we encounter the Bodhisattva Avalokiteshvara, whose name means "The one who listens deeply to the sounds of the world." The only way he is able to hear these sounds? Silence.[20]

It's all too easy to confuse solitude and loneliness, so let's take a moment to distinguish between them. Solitude occurs when someone deliberately seeks out quiet time by themselves and is a positive experience. In contrast, loneliness is a state of isolation that is typically associated with negative emotions like sadness and depression.

Creating space in one's life for idle moments of observation and appreciation is an indication you have control, instead of being a slave to continually appearing "busy" to yourself and those around you. Sure, you could go on a monastic retreat to ensure silence—but no matter how frenetic and loud your life is, I'm betting you can steal away to a quiet place for at least a little while most days or begin to observe the silent spaces between the noise of the day. I heard world renowned cellist Yo-Yo Ma once say "Music happens between the notes." Is it possible we can become sensitive enough to our surroundings as we move through the world to notice the spaces between the sounds and take solace in them?

ALIGN YOURSELF

In an interview Dan Rather did with Mother Teresa, he asked, "What do you say during your prayers?" She responded, "I listen." Dan then asked, "What does God say?" She responded, "He listens." Next time you're out for a walk or even sitting in traffic, truly listen to the rhythm of the ambient sounds you likely previously took for granted. Can you detect a pattern in surrounding birds chirping (biophony), people honking (anthrophony), or wind blowing (geophony)? Pay closer attention to the sounds and sensations inside your own body as well. It's almost like you're extending the shavasana part of a yoga class (the bit at the end when you lie down and observe your breath and body) into the rest of your day. If you pay extra close attention, you may hear the world in a more melodic way than you've ever noticed before. Imagine what a shame it would be to make it through your whole life and realize you never listened attentively enough to actually hear the music.

MOTION OF THE OCEAN

It's not just performing music that can relax us. Listening to nature's inbuilt soundtrack can have similar positive effects. I remember when a dear friend's mother was struggling with insomnia related to her arthritic pain, she bought two nature CDs—one of ocean waves lapping on the shore and another of thunderstorms—and listened to them every night before bed. The result? No more insomnia. Science shows she might have been on to something, particularly when it came to the sounds of the sea. "Slow, whooshing noises are the sounds of non-threats, which is why they work to calm people," Orfeu Buxton, an associate professor of biobehavioral health at Pennsylvania State University, told the Live Science website. "It's like they're saying: 'Don't worry, don't worry, don't worry.'"[21]

ALIGN YOURSELF

You can bring the soothing sounds of running water into your home by making a small investment in a tabletop fountain—$30 on Amazon should do the trick. Also find some soothing playlists on Spotify or, if you're old school, pick up a couple of those nature CDs I mentioned earlier at your local thrift store. Want a more versatile sonic experience? Then you could grab some Bose Sleepbuds, which come with an app that lets you select among several natural sounds and will pipe them into your ears all night to promote restful slumber.

Alignment Assignment

Notice how your posture affects your tone while communicating. You can practice with singing or humming around your house to avoid weirding anyone out. Explore vocalizing from these three positions:

1. Overextended: Your spine is arching back with your head facing upward and low back arched (Swole or Bendy archetype)
2. Collapsed Forward: Shoulders drooped forward, spine hunched, and knees collapsed inward (Mopey archetype)
3. Aligned: Standing tall in the Aligned Standing position mentioned in Chapter 6 (Aligned archetype)

CHAPTER 17

Out of Touch

"Nothing is so healing as the human touch."

—*Bobby Fischer*

Touch—often referred to as "the mother of all senses"—is foundational to human development.[1] Without it, a child will fail to thrive—meaning they won't gain weight appropriately and will literally become stunted in their physical and emotional growth. Human contact could be likened to a vital nutrient: If its effects were bottled, it would trump the impact of any performance-enhancing drug on the market.

In fact, premature infants massaged for just fifteen minutes three times a day have been shown to gain weight up to 47 percent faster than those left untouched in their incubators. Are you ready for the crazy part? The massaged infants didn't eat any more than the others! "Their weight gain seems due to the effect of contact on their metabolism," said Dr. Tiffany Field, a psychologist at the University of Miami Medical School who led the study. Dr. Field also found that human contact made the babies become more active and responsive, and they were ready to be discharged from the hospital an average of six days sooner than the infants who did not receive the daily massage.[2]

This outcome is seen across the animal kingdom, from rats to rhesus monkeys to the devastating effect on the undertouched children in Romanian orphanages in the late eighties. One potential explanation for this phenomenon comes from the late Dr. Saul Schanberg, a neuroscientist and physician, along with his fellow researchers at Duke University Department of Pharmacology. Dr. Schanberg hypothesized that touch is a part of a primitive survival system existing in all mammals. The prolonged absence of mother's touch triggers a slowing in the infant's metabolism in order to reduce its need for nourishment. In the short term this will increase likelihood of survival, but it will stunt growth if the lack of contact is prolonged.[3] He and his researchers found the touch of a mother rat licking her pups to be like an on/off switch for the growth of her offspring.

Here's the kicker: It wasn't just the care from the mother that caused the growth. The touch could be replicated by massaging the baby rats with a wet paintbrush to mimic the mother's tongue. Perhaps this is evidence that touch truly is "the *mother* of all senses."

There are innumerable factors at play in why touch is immensely valuable for physiological development, yet Western culture has been on a steady march into tactile isolation. Now let's explore the impact human contact has on our emotional life, shall we?

ALIGN YOURSELF

Try this simple and effective technique typically used to help children gain control of their emotions. It works the same way for adults and will help calm your nervous system by connecting your tactile sense with your own breath. It's called "Take Five" and can be done anywhere at any time. Whenever you're feeling a little anxious, give it a try!

1. Stretch your right palm out wide, like a star.

2. Use your left pointer finger to trace up your right thumb as you breathe in through your nose, and trace back down to the palm as you breathe out through your nose.

3. Repeat tracing up and down the rest of your fingers on your right hand until you arrive at the pinky.

4. Repeat this three to six times, and try it with your eyes closed for an even more calming effect.

EMOTIONAL INTELLIGENCE 2.0

"To touch can be to give life."

—Michelangelo

Touch is an often overlooked element of mindfulness that bridges the gap between ourselves and those around us. In a past podcast episode, my friend, the bestselling author Dr. Chris Ryan, said, "The body is the bridge to the mind." In crossing this bridge, touch is a key facilitator of the connection. When we're mindful of how we touch and are touched, we're more emotionally in tune with each other and tend to have more responsive relationships. DePauw University psychologist Matthew Hertenstein discovered we can discern the emotions of others just by touching them. This might sound a little out there, but it's true. In one study, Hertenstein and his fellow researchers asked participants to try to communicate certain emotions to a stranger who was blindfolded. Perhaps surprisingly, they were able to convey anger, fear, disgust, love, gratitude, sympathy, happiness, and sadness with up to 78 percent accuracy, solely through five seconds of touch.[4] It's worth noting the contact involved was subtle—nobody got slapped or punched in a display of anger or disgust, for example. This shows that when we're dialed in, our sense of touch is extremely sophisticated.

In another study using fMRI, scientists could see the somatosensory regions of the brain light up like a Christmas tree while the subject was being touched. They also found when the heterosexual males in the study believed they were being touched lightly on the leg by a man or woman, their brains reacted differently, suggesting social context matters when it comes to how you respond biologically to the sensation of touch.[5] We've already explored the importance of being aware of ourselves and our environment and listening intently to people, and now it seems we need to add touch-based awareness to the list of ways we can engage more deeply. Considering 55 percent of our communication is conveyed via body language, it's no surprise that physical touch plays a large part in communicating deeper-felt emotions. What can be said in silence is so much more powerful than what can be contained inside our clunky words. Embrace and cultivate this skill for optimal communication.

ALIGN YOURSELF

This may be one of the most overtly ridiculous and amazing activities I will suggest in the book to create immediate rapport, break down boundaries, and incorporate both touch and laugh therapy in your life with a group of friends. It's aptly titled "The Bread Machine," and it works like this:

1. Start with a group of at least three or four people.

2. Put one person in the middle and set a timer for two minutes (or whatever you prefer).

3. During this time the person in the middle closes their eyes, and the group kneads their arms, shoulders, legs, back, etc., as though they are a piece of dough.

4. Once the timer goes off (the bread is done), alternate the person in the middle until everyone has had a chance to receive the touch of the group.

BUILDING BONDS

"Touch comes before sight, before speech. It is the first language and the last, and it always tells the truth."

—Margaret Atwood

Atwood's insightful quote on touch being the first language and the last is literally true—it's the first sense to develop in utero and probably the most developed upon birth. It has been your primary medium of communication with the world since the beginning of "you" and very well may be the last sense you experience upon transitioning out of this body. When we're mindful about the role of touch in relationships and pay attention to its subtleties, it has a profound impact on both physical and mental well-being. To tap into this wellspring of vitality, we need to make sure we don't become cut off from face-to-face contact with others, as is becoming increasingly prevalent in our digital society. With the paradoxical disconnection of favoring online interaction over the in-person kind, we can go for days on end without hugging, holding hands, kissing, or anything of the sort—the kind of gestures that literally bind us together and make us feel whole.

Finding ways to introduce more subtle touch into our daily lives can have a profoundly positive impact, and there's some surprising evidence to back this up. Would you believe greater physical contact within sports teams is actually associated with more victories?

This was the conclusion of sociologists Michael Kraus (Yale) and Dacher Keltner (University of California, Berkeley), who did an extensive study of NBA teams and discovered a strong correlation between the total number of high fives, chest bumps and, yep, even butt slaps in each game and the team's win percentage. "Touch was associated with sophisticated metrics of higher performance at the individual and group level, and this touch to performance relationship held when accounting for player status, preseason expectations, and early season performance during the game in which touch was assessed," Kraus and Keltner concluded.[6] It's also arguable that being in a team environment compounded the positive impact of touch that the researchers noted.

If you're able to use touch appropriately and positively in a group environment, you will better align your own physical traits with the other members in the kind of emotional atmosphere you want to create. Before he took the head coaching position for the Golden State Warriors, Steve Kerr was challenged to identify one word that would encapsulate how the team played. He chose "joy." Perhaps unsurprisingly, the Warriors not only play with joyous abandon but also ranked highly in the NBA touch study as the team reaffirms their coach's mantra in how they interact and positively recognize success. The results? Three NBA championships and counting.

ALIGN YOURSELF

You might not be competing for an NBA title, but you can channel the Warriors in how you use touch thoughtfully to create a positive physical and emotional culture in any group setting. Sprinkle in more touch-based congratulations and acknowledgment of coworkers, friends, and family by offering hugs, handshakes, and high fives. If it works in the NBA to score more points, it will likely have a positive impact on your family and business, too. Start paying attention to the superpower of compassionate touch next time you're discussing a business deal, would like to express care for someone in need, or want to create a closer bond with a new friend. Take into account the quality and the frequency with which another person makes physical contact with you. A simple touch of your arm or shoulder in conversation is a key indication of rapport and trust being built.

TOUCHING TRAUMA

"The pain that you create now is always some form of non-acceptance, some form of unconscious resistance to what is."

—*Eckhart Tolle*

When someone experiences trauma, they can become hyper-sensitized to certain physical sensations, including touch. This might be because their brain's internal "pain map" has been enlarged, as in the case of a soldier injured by an IED or a civilian who's been in a car wreck, or it can be related to touch itself if somebody has been the victim of sexual abuse. While we need more scientific investigation, initial studies suggest that massage therapy can help reduce sensitivity to pain and also re-normalize pain outside the context of the initial trauma by providing a safe environment to experience appropriate and soothing touch again. A paper published in the *American Journal of Public Health* even found that massage proved beneficial to those exposed to the horrors of the 9/11 attacks.[7]

Massage can also be combined with other integrative treatments like mobility and breath work to equip the patient to tackle their symptoms when they're at home. "People who have been traumatized are no longer at home in their bodies," Pamela Fitch, the author of *Talking Body, Listening Hands*, told the American Massage Therapy Association's magazine: "Massage therapists can teach clients safe and effective ways of self-soothing and stress management."[8]

Touch also appears to have a positive impact on cardiovascular health. Research published in the fabulously named journal *Psychoneuroendocrinology* found that physical affection reduces resting heart rate, while more recent research showed open-heart surgery patients at St. Joseph's Hospital in St. Paul, Minnesota who received "healing touch" therapy before and after their procedures had shorter stays.[9] Cue a terrible pun about taking these findings to heart.

After working in the field of manual therapy for over a decade, spending literally thousands of hours in practice and seeing numerous clients relieved of emotional weight they've carried for years—I can tell you firsthand manual therapy can indeed be a powerful tool in the healing process. I believe talk therapy and manual therapy are more powerful together than they are apart and recommend seeking practitioners of both kinds who have experience working with trauma if you, a friend, or a family member are feeling overwhelmed.

ALIGN YOURSELF

Finding a trusted body worker and treating yourself to a session each month can be a great way to tap back into parts of your body that you may have disconnected from without even realizing it. If massage therapy is not your thing, I recommend exploring some form of dance as a way to wiggle out the cobwebs in the parts of your body-mind that may be more closed off. For bonus therapeutic points, journal afterward about any thoughts or feelings that came up during the massage or dance experience.

Alignment Assignment

Grab yourself a dry scrub brush and give yourself a full-body brush before you get into the shower. If dry scrub brushing isn't your thing, give yourself some slap therapy and gently tap each part of your body you're able to reach with your hands to bring more awareness to your whole self (be gentle with the more precious parts). As you're brushing or tapping, intentionally bring your awareness into the part you're touching (visualize breathing into the specific spot for added effect).

CHAPTER 18

Mindfulness—Tidy Up Your Mind to Stand Taller

"It is the mind itself which shapes the body."

—*Friedrich Schiller*

We've spent a lot of time looking at the various ways the body affects the mind, but in truth, they are indivisible processes. You can just as well come from a top-down approach by saying the state of one's mind shapes their body and be equally correct. Some people will experience greater change from a bottom-up (focus on the body to affect the mind) approach and others from a top-down (focus on the mind to affect the body); this is for you to determine for yourself. If you're not sure what works best for you, try it from both sides!

Before we go any further, it may be helpful to define "mind." I like Dr. Daniel Siegel's definition from the book *Mind*: He refers to it as an "emergent, self-organizing, embodied, and relational process that regulates the flow of energy and information." Let's repeat, it's an *embodied* and *relational* process—a continual, two-way exchange happening all the time, even right now as you're reading these words.

Lao-tzu famously said, "If you are depressed you are living in the past. If you are anxious you are living in the future. If you are at peace you are living in the present." Wise words, although he left out the postural association to thinking forward or backward. University of Aberdeen psychological scientist Lynden Miles and fellow researchers have shown that mental time travel (chromesthesia) is actually represented in the sensorimotor systems that regulate movement. They found that thinking about the past or the future literally moves the body: Focusing on the past swayed study subjects backward, while those pondering future events drifted forward! "The embodiment of time and space yields an overt behavioral marker of an otherwise invisible mental operation," explained Miles and his colleagues.[1]

This suggests perhaps the unsightly forward head posture (aka text neck) so many modern people experience could be a bigger issue than just a tight neck. Becoming more mindful creates a host of beneficial effects, ranging from pain management to releasing chronic tension, and, as we now know, improving your posture. Put simply, gaining control of your mind will allow you to become a more physically capable and resilient human being.

THE PSYCHOLOGY OF ALIGNMENT

"Happiness is not a matter of intensity, but one of balance and order and rhythm and harmony."

—*Thomas Merton*

Earlier, we touched on the link between our mood and how we carry ourselves. I'd like to return to this topic for a moment because it also pertains to this chapter's main focus: mindfulness. When you are physically aligned from head to toe, you're able to move more gracefully and powerfully. You inhabit your body more effortlessly, like what Taoist philosophers would refer to as *Wu-Wei*, which literally translates to "non-doing" and feels like effortless action.

But there's more to it than that. How we're aligned physically also has a profound impact on our mental state. We commonly think of the word "attitude" as our emotional approach to a situation, but that's a relatively modern usage. The term actually used to refer to one's physical posture. Charles Darwin, for example, described an attitude as a collection of movements such as a specific posture that depicts how a person is feeling at a particular time. Conversely, it's still common for us to talk about our "posture" toward an event in a non-bodily way, i.e., our attitude toward the event.

This isn't just a question of terminology, but also psychobiology. As discussed in to Chapter 1, such findings are backed up by the work of San Francisco State University professor of psychology Richard Peper. One of his studies found that skipping for two minutes versus walking with a slouched position noticeably changed participants' energy and hormone levels. "Emotions and thoughts affect our posture and energy levels; conversely, posture and energy affect our emotions and thoughts," Peper explained in an interview with *Fast Company*.[2]

This is why it's essential we pay attention to our physical positioning and thought life with equal care and intention. If we let either one become slouchy, it will have a significant effect on the other. When both are aligned and dynamic, we feel and act more positively. Simply put, if we want to unlock our physical potential, we must first change our minds.

EVERY MOMENT IS AN OPPORTUNITY

"Our bodies know they belong; it is our minds that make our lives so homeless."

—John O'Donoghue

It's all too easy to become stuck spinning our wheels, obsessing over what we've done and said or projecting what we're going to do next. In doing so, we fall into the trap of neglecting the value of presence, because we're stuck in a time-traveling tug-of-war between past and future. Then we clutter up any remaining space with constant social media updates, texts, and checking everything from the weather to sports scores to the news. The million-dollar question is whether we chronically check these updates because we actually care, or could it be that we've lost touch with how to be alone and present with ourselves?

Let's face it, to be completely present with yourself free of any distraction (hold that thought, I just got a text) can be uncomfortable and even scary for the uninitiated. In his book *Zen and the Art of Motorcycle Maintenance*, Robert M. Pirsig doesn't just explore what it's like to devote himself fully to fixing up an old bike. Rather, he argues that we should be fully present in everything we do, including the way we move and think. "The past cannot remember the past. The future can't generate the future," Pirsig writes. "The cutting edge of this instant right here and now is always nothing less than the totality of everything there is."[3] Think of inhabiting your mind like a training session in a gym—your thought patterns are a product of the level of care you've taken in crafting them. Each moment you practice presence by simply bringing your attention back to the here and now is like a single repetition. With time and repetitions, your presence muscle will be strong enough to sustain any distraction.

YOU ARE THE SUM OF YOUR THOUGHTS

"There is nothing either good or bad, but thinking makes it so."
—*William Shakespeare, Hamlet*

Florida State University researchers found that when participants read a couple of lines encouraging them to be mindful of every element of dishwashing—like the temperature of the water and fragrance of the dish soap—they reported a 27 percent decrease in nervousness after the task and a 25 percent increase in inspiration. You can begin doing this right now: Pay attention to the pressure of your body upon whatever it may be in contact with (chair, floor, couch, pillows, etc.). Notice the temperature on your skin, the ambient sounds, the smell of the air, the quality of light perfusing through the room, and the thoughts passing through your mind. Any time you're feeling stressed, bring your attention back to these points, and you will begin to feel calmer in your mind and body.

I've heard it said it's physically impossible to be anxious and completely present at the same time. Lessons on how to occupy the mind with ease to feel less nervous and more inspired are rarely taught in school, and the effects are evident. For example, the number of people under age twenty receiving Medicaid-funded prescriptions for antipsychotic drugs tripled between 1999 and 2008, according to an analysis by Mathematica.[4] Our thoughts are powerful and, if left unattended in the modern world, can grow out of control.

You could think of the mind like a garden with the power to yield a spectacular harvest so long as you pay it adequate attention by regularly plucking the weeds (meditation/intentional movement and breathing) so they don't choke out the nourishing plants (health/happiness/clarity). The catch with the mind garden is that it will produce whatever seed you sow, and every moment you're planting seeds that may not show themselves until next season. We think we can get away with negative self-talk and a lack of presence because we don't always see a drastic immediate change, but we don't realize the harvest of our present reality is the product of our thoughts from last season.

ALIGN YOURSELF

Pick a project for yourself and commit to a time to get started. Try to eliminate optional distractions and fully focus both body and mind on the task at hand—whether that's rebuilding an old motorcycle like Robert Pirsig or simply catching up on all those overdue household chores. And take joy in the fact that you likely have hands to wash dishes in the first place; count your blessings regularly, and the momentary magic begins poking its head out to be noticed. Realistically, you and I will both be worm food sooner than we think, so let's just consider every moment from this point forward to be extra credit; it's like icing on the cake, so enjoy it!

CLOSE OPEN LOOPS

You may have heard it said that nature abhors a vacuum. Well, it doesn't like open loops, either. Yet the attention economy we're now all part of is conspiring to open a can of loop-ass on us every single day, bombarding our brains with more new information than we can possibly hope to keep up with. Your attention is an invaluable commodity to advertisers of all kinds, and those endless notifications on your digital devices are preying on exactly that.

Every distraction grenade lobbed over your mental wall by marketers and advertisers explodes and starts a fire, as do the work-related ones that mean most white-collar workers spend 50 percent of their time receiving information rather than actually putting it to use.[5] When we let dozens, hundreds, or thousands of these blazes burn, it's no wonder we feel mentally fried at night.

Mindfulness can be the water that quells these fires and closes all those pesky open loops. As can the simple act of deliberately doing nothing. We keep buying into the delusion we have to do more, even though we know athletes who follow this dubious prescription end up injured and burned out. So just as you wouldn't do the same hard workout seven days a week, you can also give your mind a rest to process the information it's already saturated in.

UNLEASH YOUR INNER ANIMAL

Have you ever found it interesting that humans are the only creatures on the planet that "practice" meditation? We're always trying to "out-human" ourselves with hacks, shortcuts, and health fads, and yet rather than seeking man-made complexity, it could be argued that what we need to do is look to the comparative simplicity of nature for answers. One of the reasons animals don't meditate—other than their lack of intellectual development—is that the way they live every day is conducive to relaxation. Sure, they're able to trigger a self-preservatory fight-or-flight state to evade capture or to prey on food, but then they immediately down-regulate into rest-and-digest mode (not least the male lion, which sleeps up to twenty hours a day).

A single identifiable issue modern people have in relation to stress is a sincere lack of purgative tools to let go of life's daily stressors. Stanford professor and world-renowned neuroscientist Dr. Robert Sapolsky discusses the accumulative tendencies of stress in Western culture in his book *Why Zebras Don't Get Ulcers*. He points out that a distinct difference between wild animals and human beings is acute versus chronic stress. When a zebra just barely escapes the grips of a lion's jaws, it goes from full stress response, complete with a juicy cocktail of stress hormones including epinephrine (adrenaline) and cortisol, to total relaxation in a matter of moments.[6] Zebras have learned to not only accelerate their nervous system like a Tesla, but also decelerate quickly. However, we humans tend to only do the former, while neglecting the latter. As a result, we get stuck in the "on" position and never fully wind down.

This hormonal geyser we set off when we get stressed is extremely beneficial in the short term to recruit the strength and energy to react to a stimulus by increasing the heart rate, increasing blood pressure to push blood into the muscles to run, opening up the small airways in the lungs to take in as much oxygen as possible, and sharpening senses such as sight and hearing. It's like taking a race car to the track to open it up and see what it can do, a totally healthy and natural experience for the engine (occasionally). The problem arises when the gas pedal gets stuck on redline and you're attempting to pump the brakes while the throttle is still partially (or wide) open.

When we get stuck in a chronic stress state, we hold too much tension in the neck, shoulders, and upper back, often leading to headaches or migraines. We are also coiled tightly like a spring, ready to attack physically or verbally at the slightest provocation. Our vision narrows because, from an evolutionary standpoint, this stress response was engaged when a predator was nearby and our forebears had to either flee or fight. We're primed and ready for action, but often there's no outlet because we're just stuck in meetings or traffic—so we get tenser and tighter.

Perhaps *the* key lesson human beings can learn from animals is the subtle art of releasing the gas pedal. Wild animals gracefully fluctuate in between the sympathetic (gas) and parasympathetic (brake) with their natural attention to their movement and survival in nature. We possess the superpower of thinking ourselves out of a homeostatic (balanced) state. Humans tend more to sit in place and ruminate on what once was or could be. But your movement purges the stress from the body, and your attention reduces the space for it to return. We only have so much mental bandwidth; if your attention goes to mastering the way in which you pour your water or wash your car, you won't be feeding the stressful strain of thought seeds.

ALIGN YOURSELF

The next time you're feeling like you're stuck in a stressed-out state, try sitting in a sauna for twenty minutes and then taking a cold plunge. Don't have these facilities nearby? Then combining a hot and cold shower will do just fine. This will give your body a powerful reset through the autonomic nervous system and also help to clear out whatever junk is clogging up your mind.

SOUL SELF-CARE

"Your task is not to seek for love, but merely to seek and find all the barriers within yourself that you have built against it."

—*Rumi*

I've spent a lot time and energy flaying aching muscles on foam rollers, pounding them with percussion therapy guns, and rolling around on strangely shaped mobility tools. Yet I was able to resolve chronic tension I'd been poking at for years with a more inside-out approach during a Vipassana meditation retreat doing not much more than sitting in place.

When translated from the Sanskrit, *vipassana* means "to see things as they really are." The retreat involved a lot of seated meditation and focused breath work, during which we were encouraged to "scan" our bodies to discover any points holding tension and patiently allow time for them to release.

This opened my eyes to the reality that many of the chronic pains I had experienced over the years would stop flaring up if I'd just give my nervous system some time each day to quiet down. Combine this with efficient movement mechanics, along with the other principles outlined in the book, and your body is on its way to once again feeling youthful and pain-free.

This isn't merely anecdotal. Science shows us meditation can have a potent impact on reducing pain and resolving structural dysfunction. In his book *Aware*, Dr. Daniel J. Siegel cites a 10,000-person study that found those who used the Wheel of Awareness model of mindfulness reduced their chronic pain, while researchers Elizabeth Blackburn and Elissa Epel have shown that mind training boosts immune function, enhances cellular repair, and reduces inflammation. Siegel states that one of the ways practicing quiet, still self-awareness daily heals is that it puts pain back in the proper emotional context, rather than catastrophizing it. He adds that meditation is useful in "finding a way to reduce anxiety or fear and replace that with a sense of clarity or calm."[7]

ALIGN YOURSELF

Begin observing the connection between your mental state and the physical tension present in your body. Notice when you're more stressed out: Do your muscles get tighter, do your shoulders creep up to your ears, does your sphincter clench up? Is this sensation mental or physical? At what point exactly does the mental/emotional experience split from the physical, or is it all just one experience? Ponder this question for homework . . .

MIND YOUR BREATH

"Feelings come and go like clouds in a windy sky. Conscious breathing is my anchor." So said Buddhist monk Thich Nhat Hanh. His point is that no matter what he feels in response to the shifting sands of circumstance, he can always re-center himself by simply becoming aware of his breathing pattern. A lot of physical practices require you to be in a certain place to perform a set activity (like playing tennis on a court, say) or have prerequisite equipment (a basketball or soccer ball). But part of the beauty of breath work is that it's always available, you can do it anywhere, and you don't need anything other than yourself and a little self-focus.

Whether it's your mind, heart, or both surging away from you, controlled breathing provides the opportunity to play physical and cognitive catch-up. A study led by Stanford biochemists and published in *Science* showed that a certain group of nerves is in direct contact with the region of the brain that regulates arousal. There was a direct correlation between breathing depth and rate and the level of calmness or anxiousness at the neurological level.[8]

"If we can slow breathing down, as we can do by deep breathing or slow controlled breaths…these neurons then don't signal the arousal center, and don't hyperactivate the brain. So you can calm your breathing and also calm your mind," study co-author Mark Krasnow told an interviewer for *Time*.[9]

ALIGN YOURSELF

Try this breathing exercise to combine touch, breath, and mindfulness. Use the index and middle finger of your right hand to take your own pulse on your left wrist (you can find the radial artery just under the pad of your thumb on the inside of your wrist). Feel your pulse under your fingertips and begin noticing how it speeds up slightly when you breathe in and slows down as you breathe out. Simply observe this connection of your breath to your heartbeat for two to three minutes and check in with how you feel. A greater contrast in the speed of your pulse between inhalation and exhalation is an indication your body is in a balanced state.

TECHNIQUES AND RESOURCES

If you are still on the fence of all this meditation stuff and just want to dip your toes in, that's great: there are options! Here are a couple easily accessible apps I've found helpful:

- Head Space
- Waking Up: Guided Meditation with Sam Harris

Apps not your thing? No problem; let's explore a screen-free introspective practice. Chapter 13 has information on the body scan practiced upon waking in Vipassana meditation. Here is a bit more information on the actual sitting part.

VIPASSANA STYLE MEDITATION

"The cave you fear to enter holds the treasure you seek."

—Joseph Campbell

Typically, practitioners of Vipassana will sit for two total hours each day. Thankfully for you, that's not what I'm suggesting here. We're just going to borrow the basic techniques from the style and leave it up to you how long you prefer to practice. Let's try to start with setting a timer for a ten-minute sit before bed and/or upon waking.

During this time, you're going to assume a comfortable sitting position (refer to Chapter 4) and do nothing but notice the air moving through your nostrils.

Focus on the subtle sensations of the cool air moving up your airways and the warm air moving out. If this feels easy after some time, you can begin noticing any subtle sensation throughout your entire body, starting with the top of your head and slowly scanning all the way down to your toes. If that becomes easy, you can begin scanning the inside of your body for sensation. When your mind wanders (It will. A lot. That's OK.), just softly come back to the breath, free of judgment or disappointment at your mind wandering yet again.

There is a lot to this style of meditation, but that's where I'll leave it for now. Remember you can incorporate these meditation principles into your daily life, including your movement practice or gym time. Take time as often as you feel compelled to during your day to notice the sensations throughout your body and the breath moving through your nostrils (refer to Chapter 5)—you'll likely find it surprisingly calming.

For those of you interested in exploring this style of meditation in a deeper way, take a look at www.dhamma.org to read more deeply on the practice and possibly even schedule a ten-day sit for a deep-dive introduction to it. I found this experience to be invaluable and would recommend it to anyone eager to explore the uncovered nooks and crannies of their subconscious operating system (i.e., the mind).

Alignment Assignment

Make a mindfulness date with yourself to practice one of the techniques in this chapter for a few minutes every day; remember your own mindfulness spans beyond incense and meditation cushions. Start incorporating it into your movement as you walk through the world. Notice the contour of the ground under your feet, the air against your skin, and the cadence of your stride. While you're at it, start actively taking notice of the eye color of each person you come in contact with throughout your day. There are some beautiful eyes out there; enjoy!

Conclusion

"You will either step forward into growth or you will step back into safety."
—Abraham Maslow

Wow, we made it! The intention of this book is to offer easily accessible practices to seamlessly integrate optimal movement into all aspects of your daily life. This way, you can look and feel your best without depending on a single repetitive workout routine—your whole life becomes richer with opportunities to become more flexible, strong, and confident. Everything from your external environment to your internal thoughts and senses affects the way you move through the world. The principles outlined offer a full toolbox on how to begin the process of occupying your whole self in any situation that may come.

Where do we go from here, you ask? For the next month (and hopefully the rest of your life), I'd like you to actively incorporate the principles outlined in the previous chapters into your daily life until they become ingrained habits and your whole day becomes an opportunity for growth.

KEY POINTS TO ALIGN YOURSELF

Harness Your Senses

Your senses are a crucial aspect of your physical fitness. Take the tools you've learned in the Moving Your Senses section to harness the power of sight, sound, touch, and mindfulness to take control of your mental and physical state.

Take Control of Your Environment

Your environment forms your mind and body. This month, make it a priority to examine your home, office, travel, and clothing to see if they match your ideal vision for your future self. If your environments are forming your body into a sub-optimal position, it's about time you Align them!

FIVE DAILY MOVEMENT PRINCIPLES

Each of the daily movements mentioned in Part II have the power to provide you with more strength and ease in living in the short term and grant you physical autonomy into the final days with your body in the long run. As mentioned in Chapter 4, no human needs to go through the "I've fallen and I can't get up" moment as an elderly person if they follow the principles outlined below! This month make a point to:

- Spend at least thirty total minutes on the ground (tag #floorculture to share with the Align Community).
- Hang for a total of ninety seconds to three minutes per day.
- Hinge from your hips in most household and work activities.
- Breathe almost entirely through your nose during the day and night.
- Make more excuses for yourself to take walks each day (park further away from your destination, take walk breaks while working, schedule walk meetings, take your calls while walking outside, etc.) and pay attention while doing so, like a moving meditation.

CLOSING THOUGHTS

Perhaps the most valuable—and yet all too often overlooked—element of optimal health and movement function is determining your reason to move in the first place. Those mindful folks responsible for the rich Japanese language came up with a convenient term for this: *ikigai*. This translates to your "reason for being." At the end of the day, if you don't have a good *ikigai*, colors will seem less bright, flavors less flavorful, relationships less meaningful, and your posture less upright. Fill yourself with purpose by devoting more of your time to service free of expectations, and you'll experience postural change a foam roller could never deliver.

Remember, there's no pause on your self-development, and there's no need to wait for a yoga class or gym to work on your fitness: You're continually in a state of construction, no matter where you are or what time it is. You can use this book as a roadmap leading you back to a state of balance. Then, the ultimate step for true alignment is letting go of the rules and stepping into your own natural way of being. You will only find your ideal postures in sitting, standing, laying, walking, and breathing when you stop fixating on what "perfect" should look like and start listening to what your body has known all along.

Finally, I'll leave us with the words of Dr. Andrew Taylor Still, the founder of osteopathy: "Harmony only dwells where obstructions do not exist." Make each day a process of dropping restrictions on your capacity to give and receive love—our time in these bodies is far too short to limp through with a guarded heart. If these are your priorities, you're set to *move* well in your life.

It's been my pleasure and honor to bring this collection of ideas to you. Thanks for coming along for the ride.

Notes

You can find your own digital workbook—including how I incorporate each chapter's recommendations into my own daily life and how you can form them to meet your specific goals—at www.TheAlignBook.com.

Chapter 1: Stand Up for Yourself—Posture and Personality

1. Pablo Brunol et al., "Body Posture Effects on Self-Evaluation: A Self-Validation Approach," *European Journal of Social Psychology*, August 2009, available online at https://onlinelibrary.wiley.com/doi/abs/10.1002/ejsp.607.
2. Lisa Owens Viani, "Good Posture Is Important for Physical and Mental Health," *SF State News*, December 2017, available online at https://news.sfsu.edu/news-story/good-posture-important-physical-and-mental-health.
3. Bessel van der Kolk, *The Body Keeps the Score* (New York: Penguin, 2015), 112.
4. Peter Levine, *Waking the Tiger* (Berkeley, CA: North Atlantic Books, 1997), 95.
5. "The Economic Impact of the Coffee Industry," National Coffee Association, available online at http://www.ncausa.org/Industry-Resources/Economic-Impact.
6. Dana R. Carney, Amy Cuddy, and A. J. Nap, "Power Posing: Brief Nonverbal Displays Affect Neuroendocrine Levels and Risk Tolerance," *Psychological Science,* September 2010, available online at http://www.people.hbs.edu/acuddy/in%20press,%20carney,%20cuddy,%20&%20yap,%20psych%20science.pdf.
7. Amy Cuddy, "Your Body Language May Shape Who You Are," TED Talks, available online at https://www.ted.com/talks/amy_cuddy_your_body_language_shapes_who_you_are?language=en.
8. Joseph P. Simmons, Uri Simonsohn, "Power Posing: P-curving the Evidence" (2017) *Psychological Science*, 28 (5), 687–693. Available online at https://journals.sagepub.com/doi/abs/10.1177/0956797616658563?journalCode=pssa.
9. Amy J. C. Cuddy, S. Jack Schultz, Nathan E. Fosse, "P-Curving a More Comprehensive Body of Research on Postural Feedback Reveals Clear Evidential Value for Power-Posing Effects: Reply to Simmons and Simonsohn" (2017). *Psychological Science*,

29(4), 656–666. Available online at https://journals.sagepub.com/eprint/CzbNAn7 Ch6ZZirK9yMGH/full.

10. Jeff Thompson, "Is Nonverbal Communication a Numbers Game?," *Psychology Today*, September 2011, available online at https://www.psychologytoday.com/us/blog/beyond -words/201109/is-nonverbal-communication-numbers-game.

11. Albert Mehrabian, *Nonverbal Communication* (Piscataway, NJ: 1972), 108.

12. Chuck Hustmyre and Jay Dixit, "Marked for Mayhem," *Psychology Today*, January 2009, available online at https://www.psychologytoday.com/us/articles/200901/marked-mayhem.

13. Dr. Paul Ekman, "Are There Universal Facial Expressions?," available online at https:// www.paulekman.com/resources/universal-facial-expressions.

14. Andreas Hennenlotter et al. "The Link Between Facial Feedback and Neural Activity within Central Circuits of Emotion—New Insights from Botulinum Toxin–Induced Denervation of Frown Muscles," *Cerebral Cortex* 19:3, March 2009, 537–542, https:// doi.org/10.1093/cercor/bhn104.

15. Ibid.

16. R. J. Larsen, "Facilitating the Furrowed Brow: An Unobtrusive Test of the Facial Feed-back Hypothesis Applied to Unpleasant Affect," *Cognition and Emotion* 6(5) (September 1992): 321–33, https://www.ncbi.nlm.nih.gov/pubmed/29022461.

Chapter 2: Rigidity Tends to Break—Play May Save Your Brain and Body

1. Richard W. Byrne, "The What as Well as the Why of Animal Fun," *Current Biology*, January 2015, available online at https://www.cell.com/current-biology/comments /S0960-9822(14)01123-3.

2. "Less-Structured Time in Children's Daily Lives Predicts Self-Directed Executive Functioning," *Frontiers in Psychology*, June 2014, available online at https://www.fron tiersin.org/articles/10.3389/fpsyg.2014.00593/full.

3. Jaak Panksepp et al., "A Novel NMDA Receptor Glycine-site Partial Agonist, GLYX-13, Has Therapeutic Potential for the Treatment of Autism," *Neuroscience & Biobehavioral Reviews*, 2011, available online at https://doi.org/10.1016/j.neubiorev.2011.06.006.

4. Stuart Brown, *Play: How it Shapes the Brain, Opens the Imagination, and Invigorates the Soul* (New York: Avery, 2009), 41.

5. M. Bronikowska et al., "You Think You Are Too Old to Play? Playing Games and Aging," *Human Movement*, available online at https://www.degruyter.com/downloadpdf /j/humo.2011.12.issue-1/v10038-010-0030-2/v10038-010-0030-2.pdf.

6. Patricia J. Holhbein, "The Power of Play in Developing Emotional Intelligence Impact-ing Leadership Success: A Study of the Leadership Team in a Midwest Private, Liberal Arts University," Pepperdine University, June 2015, available online at https://search

.proquest.com/openview/792ae392ff6d43e60b0914c3ad539f2f/1?pq-origsite=gschola r&cbl=18750&diss=y; B. Janet Hibbs and Anthony Rostain, "Why 90 Percent of Generation Z Says They're Stressed Out," *Psychology Today*, December 2018, available online at https://www.psychologytoday.com/us/blog/the-stressed-years-their-lives/201812 /why-90-percent-generation-z-says-theyre-stressed-out.

7. Cale D. Magnusson and Lynn A. Barnett, "The Playful Advantage: How Playfulness Enhances Coping with Stress," *Leisure Sciences*, March 2013, available online at https:// www.tandfonline.com/doi/abs/10.1080/01490400.2013.761905?journalCode=ulsc20.

8. Ibid.

9. Stephen Porges, "Play as a Neural Exercise: Insights into Polyvagal Theory," The Power of Play for Mind-Brain Health, Mindgains.org, available online at https://mindgains .org/bonus/GAINS-The-Power-of-Play-for-Mind-Brain-Health.pdf.

Chapter 3: Tools and Techniques to Align Your Body

1. R. Schleip et al., "Active Fascial Contractility: Fascia May Be Able to Contract in a Smooth Muscle-Like Manner and Thereby Influence Musculoskeletal Dynamics," *Medical Hypothesis*, 2005, available online at https://www.ncbi.nlm.nih.gov/pubmed/15922099.

2. H. M. Langevin et al., "Mechanical Signaling Through Connective Tissue: A Mechanism for the Therapeutic Effect of Acupuncture," *FASEB Journal*, October 2001, available online at https://www.ncbi.nlm.nih.gov/pubmed/11641255.

3. Andrew Still, *Philosophy of Osteopathy* (independently published via lulu.com, 2018), 18.

4. Sahib S. Khalsa et al., "Interoception and Mental Health: A Roadmap," *Biological Psychiatry. Cognitive Neuroscience and Neuroimaging*, June 2018, available online at https:// www.ncbi.nlm.nih.gov/pmc/articles/PMC6054486/.

5. Brian C. Clark et al., "The Power of the Mind: The Cortex as a Critical Determinant of Muscle Strength/Weakness," *Journal of Neurophysiology*, December 2014, available online at https://www.physiology.org/doi/full/10.1152/jn.00386.2014.

6. Kai J. Miller et al., "Cortical Activity During Motor Execution, Motor Imagery, and Imagery-Based Online Feedback," *PNAS*, March 2010, available online at https://www .pnas.org/content/107/9/4430; Vinoth K. Ranganathan et al., "From Mental Power to Muscle Power—Gaining Strength by Using the Mind," *Neuropsychologia*, 2004, available online at https://www.sciencedirect.com/science/article/pii/S002839320300325.7.

Chapter 4: Floor Sitting: Your Foundation for Self-Care

1. Leonardo Barbosa, Barreto de Brito, et al., "Ability to Sit and Rise from the Floor as a Predictor of All-Cause Mortality," *Preventive Cardiology,* 2012, available online at http://geriatrictoolkit.missouri.edu/srff/deBrito-Floor-Rise-Mortality-2012.pdf.

2. "Falls Prevention Facts," *National Council on Aging*, available online at https://www .ncoa.org/news/resources-for-reporters/get-the-facts/falls-prevention-facts/.

3. Phillip Beach, *Muscles and Meridians* (London: Churchill Livingstone, 2010), 134.

4. Wang Xi et al., "Material Approaches to Active Tissue Dynamics," *Nature*, December 2018, available online at https://www.nature.com/articles/s41578-018-0066-z.

5. A. D. Woolf and B. Pfleger, "Burden of Major Musculoskeletal Conditions," *Bulletin of the World Health Organization*, 2003, available online at https://www.ncbi.nlm.nih.gov /pubmed/14710506; "The Cost of Arthritis in US Adults," *CDC*, available online at https://www.cdc.gov/arthritis/data_statistics/cost.htm.

6. James A. Levine, "The "NEAT Defect" in "Human Obesity: The Role of Nonexercise Activity Thermogenesis," *Endocrinology Update*, 2007, available online at https://www .mayoclinic.org/documents/mc5810-0307-pdf/doc-20079082.

7. Christopher Shea, "Mindful Exercise, *New York Times*, December 2007, https://www .nytimes.com/2007/12/09/magazine/09mindfulexercise.html.

8. James A. Levine, "The "NEAT Defect" in Human Obesity: The Role of Nonexercise Activity Thermogenesis," *Endocrinology Update,* 2007, available online at https://www .mayoclinic.org/documents/mc5810-0307-pdf/doc-20079082.

Chapter 5: Nasal Breathing: Tuning Your Engine

1. H. R. Colten and B. M. Altevogt, "Sleep Disorders and Sleep Deprivation: An Unmet Public Health Problem," Institute of Medicine (US) Committee on Sleep Medicine and Research, 2006, available online at https://www.ncbi.nlm.nih.gov/pubmed/20669438.

2. Emma M. Seppälä, Jack B. Nitschke, Dana L. Tudorascu, et al., "Breathing-Based Meditation Decreases Posttraumatic Stress Disorder Symptoms in U.S. Military Veterans: A Randomized Controlled Longitudinal Study," *Journal of Traumatic Stress*, 2014, available online at https://onlinelibrary.wiley.com/doi/full/10.1002/jts.21936.

3. I. M. Lin et al., "Breathing at a Rate of 5.5 Breaths per Minute with Equal Inhalation-to-Exhalation Ratio Increases Heart Rate Variability," *International Journal of Psychophysiology*, March 2014, available online at https://www.ncbi.nlm.nih.gov/pubmed/24380741.

4. Sandra Kahn and Robert R. Erlich, *Jaws: The Story of a Hidden Epidemic* (Palo Alto, CA: Stanford University Press, 2018), 6.

5. Alex Hutchinson, *Endure* (New York: William Morrow, 2017), 121–122.

6. J. Key, "'The core': Understanding it, and retraining its dysfunction," *Journal of Bodywork & Movement Therapies*, 2013, available online at http://dx.doi.org/10.1016/j.jbmt .2013.03.012.

Chapter 6: Hip Hinging: Give Me Leverage and I'll Move the World

1. "Morihei Ueshiba," *The Art of Peace* (Boulder, CO: Shambala, 2007), 35.

2. Esther Gokhale, *8 Steps to a Pain-Free Back: Natural Posture* (Pendo Press, 2008), 21.

3. K. K. Hansraj, "Assessment of Stresses in the Cervical Spine Caused by Posture and Position of the Head," *Surgical Technology International*, available online at https://www.ncbi.nlm.nih.gov/pubmed/25393825.

4. Jonathan Kingdon, *Lowly Origin: Where, When, and Why Our Ancestors First Stood Up* (Princeton, NJ: Princeton University Press, 2003), 19.

5. Dr. Kelly Starrett and Glen Cordoza, *Becoming a Supple Leopard*, 2nd edition (Las Vegas: Victory Belt, 2015), 15.

6. Stuart McGill, "Hip Anatomy," OTP Books, available online at https://www.otpbooks.com/stuart-mcgill-hip-anatomy/.

Chapter 7: Hanging: The Power of Decompression

1. Richard Gray, "The Real Reasons Why We Walk on Two Legs, and Not Four," BBC, December 2016, available online at http://www.bbc.com/earth/story/20161209-the-real-reasons-why-we-walk-on-two-legs-and-not-four.

2. Wynne Parry, "Exaptation: How Evolution Uses What's Available," Live Science, September 2013, available online at https://www.livescience.com/39688-exaptation.html; Brian G. Richmond et al., "Origin of Human Bipedalism: The Knuckle-Walking Hypothesis Revisited," *Yearbook of Physical Anthropology*, 2001, available online at http://users.clas.ufl.edu/krigbaum/proseminar/richmond_etal_2001_ypa.pdf.

3. Robert Jurmain et al., *Essentials of Physical Anthropology*, 7th edition (Boston: Cengage Learning, 2008), 109

4. John Kirsch, *Shoulder Pain?* (Morgan, NC: Bookstand Publishing, 2013), 6–7.

5. Kristina Killgrove, "Brawny Bones Reveal Medieval Hungarian Warriors Were Accomplished Archers," *Forbes*, September 2015, available online at https://www.forbes.com/sites/kristinakillgrove/2015/09/30/brawny-bones-reveal-10th-century-hungarian-warriors-were-accomplished-archers/#10f1c4a35f71.

6. John Gribbin and Jeremy Cherfas, *The First Chimpanzee*, 2nd Edition (New York: Penguin Science, 2001), 10.

7. W. H. Irwin McClean, "Genetic Disorders of Palm Skin and Nail," *Journal of Anatomy*, 2003, available online at https://www.ncbi.nlm.nih.gov/pmc/articles/PMC1571049/.

8. Howard LeWine, "Grip Strength May Provide Clues to Heart Health," Harvard Health Publishing, May 2015, available online at https://www.health.harvard.edu/blog/grip-strength-may-provide-clues-to-heart-health-201505198022.

9. E. Fain and C. Weatherford, "Comparative Study of Millennials' (Age 20–34 Years) Grip and Lateral Pinch with the Norms," *Journal of Hand Therapy*, available online at https://www.ncbi.nlm.nih.gov/pubmed/26869476.

10. Salim Yusuf and Koon Teo, "PURE—Prospective Urban and Rural Epidemiological Study," *CoHeart*, available online at http://www.coheart.ca/projects/pure; "Chronic Low Back Pain on the Rise: UNC Study Finds 'Alarming Increase' in Prevalence," 2009, UNC School of Medicine, available online at http://www.med.unc.edu/www/newsarchive/2009/february/chronic-low-back-pain-on-the-rise-unc-study-finds-alarming-increase-in-prevalence.

11. Pavel Tsatsouline, *Relax into Stretch* (St. Paul, MN: Dragon Door Publications, 2001), 3–4.

12. Gray Cook, "Hitting Save on a Movement Document," September 24, 2015, *Functional Movement*, available online at https://www.functionalmovement.com/articles/FMS%20Video%20Series/640/hitting_save_on_a_movement_document.

Chapter 8: Walking: Circulating Your Mind and Body

1. Dan Buettner, *The Blue Zones, Second Edition: 9 Lessons for Living Longer from the People Who've Lived the Longest* (New York: National Geographic, 2012), 63.

2. Stacy Simon, "Study: Even a Little Daily Walking May Help You Live Longer," American Cancer Society, October 19, 2017, available online at https://www.cancer.org/latest-news/study-even-a-little-walking-may-help-you-live-longer.html.

3. Craig Stanford, *Upright* (Boston: Houghton Mifflin, 2003), xix.

4. Ibid., 166–170.

5. Robert E. Shadwick, "Elastic Energy Storage in Tendons: Mechanical Differences Related to Function and Age," *Journal of Applied Physiology*, 1995, available online at https://pdfs.semanticscholar.org/9cb2/fe7d04a2fafe5c550f5845c37eb43fe89e8f.pdf (page 1033).

6. Steven Levy, "One More Thing: Inside Apple's Insanely Great (Or Just Insane) New Mothership," *Wired*, May 16, 2017, available online at https://www.wired.com/2017/05/apple-park-new-silicon-valley-campus.

7. E. Sng, E. Frith, and P. D. Loprinzi, "Temporal Effects of Acute Walking Exercise on Learning and Memory Function," *American Journal of Health Promotion*, September 2018, available online at https://www.ncbi.nlm.nih.gov/pubmed/29284283.

8. Kirk I. Erickson et al., "Exercise Training Increases Size of Hippocampus and Improves Memory," *Proceedings of the National Academy of Sciences* 108 (7): 3017–3022, available online at http://www.pnas.org/content/early/2011/01/25/1015950108.

9. Michael A. Yappa, "Hippocampus," *Encyclopedia Britannica*, available online at https://www.britannica.com/science/hippocampus.

10. Marily Oppezzo and Daniel L. Schwartz, "Give Your Ideas Some Legs: The Positive

Effect of Walking on Creative Thinking," *Journal of Experimental Psychology: Learning, Memory, and Cognition,* 2014, available online at https://www.apa.org/pubs/journals/releases/xlm-a0036577.pdf.

11. Heidi Godman, "Regular Exercise Changes the Brain to Improve Memory, Thinking Skills," *Harvard Health,* April 9, 2014, available online at https://www.health.harvard.edu/blog/regular-exercise-changes-brain-improve-memory-thinking-skills-201404097110.

12. C. H. Hillman, "The Effect of Acute Treadmill Walking on Cognitive Control and Academic Achievement in Preadolescent Children," *Neuroscience,* March 2010, available online at https://www.ncbi.nlm.nih.gov/pmc/articles/PMC2667807/.

13. Eben Weiss, "The Art of Wayfinding," *Outside,* April 4, 2018, available online at https://www.outsideonline.com/2294891/art-wayfinding.

14. Lin Edwards, "Study Suggests Reliance on GPS May Reduce Hippocampus Function as We Age," *Medical Xpress,* November 2010, available online at https://medicalxpress.com/news/2010-11-reliance-gps-hippocampus-function-age.html;

15. David Dobbs, "Are GPS Apps Messing with Our Brains?," *Mother Jones,* November 2016, available online at https://www.motherjones.com/media/2016/11/gps-brain-function-memory-navigation-maps-apps.

16. Katy Bowman, "13 Ways to Make Your Walk More Nutritious," *Nutritious Movement,* available online at https://www.nutritiousmovement.com/13-ways-to-make-your-walk-more-nutritious/.

17. Phillip Beach, *Muscles and Meridians* (London: Churchill Livingstone, 2010), 145.

18. S. Beddhu et al., "Light-Intensity Physical Activities and Mortality in the United States General Population and CKD Subpopulation," *Clinical Journal of the American Society of Nephrology,* July 2015, available online at https://www.ncbi.nlm.nih.gov/pubmed/25931456.

19. "Physical Activity, Any Type or Amount, Cuts Health Risk from Sitting," Science Daily, January 2019, available online at https://www.sciencedaily.com/releases/2019/01/190114170601.htm

Chapter 9: Clothing—If the Shoe Fits

1. J. Flensmark, "Is There an Association Between the Use of Heeled Footwear and Schizophrenia?," *Medical Hypothesis,* 2001, available online at https://www.ncbi.nlm.nih.gov/pubmed/15325026.

Chapter 10: Align Your Home for Optimal Health and Creativity

1. Alison Abbot, "City Living Marks the Brain," *Nature,* June 2011, available online at https://www.nature.com/news/2011/110622/full/474429a.html.

2. "How Does the Brain's Spatial Map Change When We Change the Shape of the Room?," University College London, March 2018, available online at https://www.ucl.ac.uk/swc/sainsbury-wt-news-pub/how-does-the-brains-spatial-map-change-when-we-change-the-shape-of-the-room.

3. Kashmira Gander, "How Architecture Uses Space, Light, and Material to Affect Your Mood," *The Independent*, April 2016, available online at https://www.independent.co.uk/life-style/design/how-architecture-uses-space-light-and-material-to-affect-your-mood-american-institute-architects-a6985986.html.

4. Amber Brooks and Leon Lack, "A Brief Afternoon Nap Following Nocturnal Sleep Restriction: Which Nap Duration is Most Recuperative?," *Sleep,* June 2006, available online at https://academic.oup.com/sleep?pid=26564; Linh Nguyen, "Science Says This Is Exactly How to Nap to Be at Your Best," *Forbes*, June 2016, available online at https://www.forbes.com/sites/quora/2016/06/24/science-says-this-is-exactly-how-to-nap-to-be-at-your-best/#602ff7e677de.

5. Sara Mednick, *Take a Nap! Change Your Life.* (New York: Workman, 2006), 139.

Chapter 11: Aligning Your Office for Better Movement

1. "American Time Use Survey," US Department of Labor, available online at https://www.bls.gov/tus/charts.htm.

2. Matthew A. Davis, "Where the United States Spends Its Spine Dollars: Expenditures on Different Ambulatory Services for the Management of Back and Neck Conditions," *Spine*, September 2013, available online at https://www.ncbi.nlm.nih.gov/pmc/articles/PMC3423501/.

3. Robert Ulrich, "View through a Window May Influence Recovery from Surgery," *Science,* 1984, available online at http://science.sciencemag.org/content/224/4647/420.

4. Slepian, M. L., & Ambady, N. "Fluid movement and creativity," *Journal of Experimental Psychology: General*, November 2012. Retrieved from https://www.ncbi.nlm.nih.gov/pubmed/22352395.

5. Keith Bryant, "Rounded Corners and Why They Are Here to Stay," *Design Modo*, available online at https://designmodo.com/rounded-corners/.

6. Jennifer Wallace, "Why It's Good for Grown-Ups to Go Play," *Washington Post*, May 20, 2017, available online at https://www.washingtonpost.com/national/health-science/why-its-good-for-grown-ups-to-go-play/2017/05/19/99810292-fd1f-11e6-8ebe-6e0dbe4f2bca_story.html?noredirect=on&utm_term=.3f4807948e65.

7. A. Cogoli, "Changes Observed in Lymphocyte Behavior During Gravitational Unloading," *ASGSB Bulletin*, July 1991, available online at https://www.ncbi.nlm.nih.gov/pubmed/11537173.

Chapter 12: Therapeutic Movement for Driving and Travel

1. "Americans Spend an Average of 17,600 Minutes Driving Each Year," AAA, September 2016, available online at https://newsroom.aaa.com/2016/09/americans-spend-average-17600-minutes-driving-year/.

2. C. Hoehner et al., "Commuting Distance, Cardiorespiratory Fitness, and Metabolic Risk," *American Journal of Preventative Medicine*, June 2012, available online at https://www.ajpmonline.org/article/S0749-3797(12)00167-5/abstract.

3. "Commuting and Personal Well-being, 2014," Office for National Statistics, February 2014, available online at https://webarchive.nationalarchives.gov.uk/20160105231823/http://www.ons.gov.uk/ons/rel/wellbeing/measuring-national-well-being/commuting-and-personal-well-being—2014/art-commuting-and-personal-well-being.html

4. N. Babault et al., "Activation of Human Quadriceps Femoris During Isometric, Concentric, and Eccentric Contractions," *Journal of Applied Physiology*, December 2001, available online at https://www.ncbi.nlm.nih.gov/pubmed/11717228.

5. "An Ancient Medical Treasure at Your Fingertips," available online at https://wayback.archive-it.org/org-350/20180911192432/https://www.nlm.nih.gov/news/turn_page_egyptian.html.

6. "Data and Statistics on Venous Thromboembolism," CDC, available online at https://www.cdc.gov/ncbddd/dvt/data.html.

Chapter 13: The Aligned Morning—How to Start Your Day Upright

1. "A Brief History of Salt," *Time,* March 1982, available online at http://content.time.com/time/magazine/article/0,9171,925341,00.html.

2. Cheryl L. Laffer, "Is Sodium Restriction Important to Hypertension?," *Medscape*, January 2019, available online at https://www.medscape.com/viewarticle/480719_2.

3. H. C. Sherman and A. O. Gettler, "The Balance of Acid Forming and Base Forming Elements in Foods, and Its Relation to Ammonia Metabolism," *Journal of Biological Chemistry,* 1912, available online at http://www.jbc.org/content/11/4/323.full.pdf.

4. Joseph Cafone, "Disruption to the Circadian Rhythm Can Cause Weight Gain, Study Says," ABC News, April 2018, available online at https://abcnews.go.com/Health/disruption-circadian-rhythm-weight-gain-study/story?id=54202080.

5. Robert Emmons and Michael McCullough, "Counting Blessings Versus Burdens: An Experimental Investigation of Gratitude and Subjective Well-Being in Daily Life," *Journal of Personality and Social Psychology*, 2003, available online at https://greatergood.berkeley.edu/images/application_uploads/Emmons-CountingBlessings.pdf.

6. Rollin McCraty, "The Appreciative Heart: The Psychophysiology of Appreciation,"

January 2002, available online at https://www.researchgate.net/publication/232478613 _The_Appreciative_Heart_The_Psychophysiology_of_Appreciation.

7. C. L. Flinchbaugh et al., "Student well-being interventions: The effects of stress management techniques and gratitude journaling in the management education classroom," *Journal of Management Education*, 2012, available online at https://journals.sagepub.com /doi/abs/10.1177/1052562911430062.

8. K. M. Krpan et al., "An everyday activity as a treatment for depression: the benefits of expressive writing for people diagnosed with major depressive disorder," *Journal of Affective Disorders* 150(3) (2013): 1148–1151, available online at https://www.ncbi.nlm.nih.gov /pubmed/23790815

9. Robert Emmons and Michael McCullough, "Counting Blessings Versus Burdens: An Experimental Investigation of Gratitude and Subjective Well-Being in Daily Life," *Journal of Personality and Social Psychology*, 2003, available online at https://greatergood .berkeley.edu/images/application_uploads/Emmons-CountingBlessings.pdf.

10. N. A. Shevchuk, "Adapted Cold Shower as a Potential Treatment for Depression," *Medical Hypothesis*, 2008, available online at https://www.ncbi.nlm.nih.gov/pubmed /17993252.

11. Chantal Moret and Mike Briley, "The Importance of Norepinephrine in Depression," *Neuropsychiatric Disease and Treatment,* 2011, available online at https://www.ncbi.nlm .nih.gov/pmc/articles/PMC3131098/.

Chapter 14: The Aligned Evening—Accessing the Superpowers of Sleep

1. Anahad O'Connor, "The Claim: Lying on Your Left Side Eases Heartburn," *New York Times*, October 2010, available online at https://www.nytimes.com/2010/10/26/health/26really .html.

2. Kristen Domonell, "What Sleeping Position Is Best for You?," CNN, March 2017, available online at https://www.cnn.com/2016/03/18/health/sleep-positions-good-bad/index .html.

3. H. Lee et al., "The Effect of Body Posture on Brain Glymphatic Transport," *Journal of Neuroscience*, August 2015, available online at http://www.jneurosci.org/content/35/31/11034 .short.

4. J. R. Davidson et al., "Growth Hormone and Cortisol Secretion in Relation to Sleep and Wakefulness," *Journal of Psychiatry and Neuroscience,* July 1991, available online at https://www.ncbi.nlm.nih.gov/pmc/articles/PMC1188300/.

5. Saffron Alexander, "Why You Shouldn't Eat Late at Night, According to Science," *The Telegraph*, June 2017, available online at https://www.telegraph.co.uk/health-fitness /body/shouldnt-eat-late-night-according-science/.

6. Cibele Aparecida Crispim et al., "Relationship between Food Intake and Sleep Pattern in Healthy Individuals," *Journal of Clinical Sleep Medicine*, 2011, available online at http://jcsm.aasm.org/viewabstract.aspx?pid=28375.

7. Valter D. Longo and Satchidananda Panda, "Fasting, circadian rhythms, and time restricted feeding in healthy lifespan," *Cell Metabolism*, 2017, available online at https://www.ncbi.nlm.nih.gov/pubmed/27304506.

8. S.O. Quaswari et al., "The effect of intermittent fasting during Ramadan on sleep, sleepiness, cognitive function, and circadian rhythm," *Sleep & Breath*, 2017, available online at https://www.ncbi.nlm.nih.gov/pubmed/28190167.

9. Thomas Cronin, "Seeing Without Eyes," *Scientific American*, August 2017, available online at https://www.scientificamerican.com/article/seeing-without-eyes1/.

10. Kenji Obayashi et al., "Bedroom Light Exposure at Night and the Incidence of Depressive Symptoms: A Longitudinal Study of the HEIJO-KYO Cohort," *American Journal of Epidemiology*, July 2017, available online at https://academic.oup.com /aje/article-abstract/187/3/427/4056592?redirectedFrom=fulltext.

11. "Sleeping with artificial light at night associated with weight gain in women," National Institutes of Health, June 2019, available online at https://www.nih.gov/news-events /news-releases/sleeping-artificial-light-night-associated-weight-gain-women.

Chapter 15: Near Sight—Your Eyes Need Movement, Too!

1. João Medeiro, "Our Obsession with Phones Could Be Changing the Shape of Our Eyes," *Wired*, available online at https://www.wired.co.uk/article/eye-sight.

2. Niraj Chokshi, "Out of the Office: More People Are Working Remotely, Survey Finds," *New York Times,* February 15, 2017.

3. Joseph Mercola, "How LED Lighting May Compromise Your Health," October 2013, available online at https://articles.mercola.com/sites/articles/archive/2016/10/23/near -infrared-led-lighting.aspx.

4. Andrew Huberman, Instagram posts between February 8 and 14, 2019, available online at https://www.instagram.com/hubermanlab/.

5. Magdalena M. H. E. van der Berg et al., "Modulation of Attentional Inhibition by Norepinephrine and Cortisol after Psychological Stress," *International Journal of Environmental Research and Public Health*, December 2015.

6. Bamini Gopinath et al., "Influence of Physical Activity and Screen Time on the Retinal Microvasculature in Young Children," *Arteriosclerosis, Thrombosis, and Vascular Biology*, May 2011, available online at https://www.ahajournals.org/doi/full/10.1161/atvbaha .110.219451.

7. Morgan Childs, "A Week of Darkness, for Your Health," *The Atlantic,* July 2018, available

online at https://www.theatlantic.com/health/archive/2018/07/darkness-therapy-czech
-republic/564365/.

8. Anette Kjellgren and Jessica Westman, "Beneficial Effects of Treatment with Sensory
Isolation in Flotation-Tank as a Preventive Health-Care Intervention—A Randomized
Controlled Pilot Trial," *BMC Complementary and Alternative Medicine*, October 2014,
available online at https://www.ncbi.nlm.nih.gov/pmc/articles/PMC4219027/.

9. "Smartphone Use: Distracted Pedestrians Walk Slower and Are Less Steady on Their
Feet," Science Daily, July 2018, available online at https://www.sciencedaily.com
/releases/2018/07/180731125546.htm

10. Takahiro Higuchi, "Visuomotor Control of Human Adaptive Locomotion: Understanding the Anticipatory Nature," *Frontiers in Psychology*, 2013, available online at
https://www.ncbi.nlm.nih.gov/pmc/articles/PMC3655271/.

11. Amanda Johnson, "Florence Williams Wants You to Get More Nature in Your Life,"
Standard-Examiner, October 2018, available online at https://www.standard.net/enter
tainment/arts/florence-williams-wants-you-to-get-more-nature-in-your/article
_b85b416a-a8fd-5bae-992e-9242cd5028ba.html.

12. Richard Louv, *Vitamin N* (Chapel Hill, NC: Algonquin Books, 2016), 27.

Chapter 16: Finding Your Voice—the Way Sound Moves Us

1. Steve Connor, "Human Brain Has Dedicated Set of Nerve Cells That Respond Only
to Sound of Music, Study Finds," *The Independent*, available online at https://www
.independent.co.uk/news/science/human-brain-has-dedicated-set-of-nerve-cells
-that-respond-only-to-sound-of-music-study-finds-a6780246.html.

2. R. C. Kessler et al., "Posttraumatic stress disorder in the National Comorbidity Survey," *Archives of General Psychiatry*, 1995, available online at https://www.ncbi.nlm.nih
.gov/pubmed/7492257.

3. Nora Landis-Shack, Adrienne J. Heinz, and Marcel O. Bonn-Miller, "Music Therapy
for Posttraumatic Stress in Adults: A Theoretical Review," *Psychomusicology*, December
2017, available online at https://www.ncbi.nlm.nih.gov/pmc/articles/PMC5744879/.

4. Myriam V. Thoma et al., "The Effect of Music on the Human Stress Response," *PLoS One*,
2013, available online at https://www.ncbi.nlm.nih.gov/pmc/articles/PMC3734071/.

5. A. J. Blood and R. J. Satorre, "Intensely Pleasurable Responses to Music Correlate
with Activity in Brain Regions Implicated in Reward and Emotion," *Proceedings of the
National Academy of Sciences*, September 2001, available online at https://www.ncbi.nlm
.nih.gov/pubmed/11573015/.

6. Maria Sorensen, "The Neurology of Music for Post-Traumatic-Stress Disorder Treatment:
A Theoretical Approach for Social Work Implications," February 2015, St. Catherine

University of St. Thomas, available online at https://sophia.stkate.edu/cgi/viewcontent .cgi?article=1526&context=msw_papers.

7. Deb A. Dana, *The Polyvagal Theory in Therapy* (New York: W.W. Norton, 2018), 113.

8. J. R. Keeler, "The Neurochemistry and Social Flow of Singing: Bonding and Oxyto-cin," *Frontiers of Human Neuroscience*, September 2015, available online at https://www .ncbi.nlm.nih.gov/pmc/articles/PMC4585277/.

9. Bangalore G. Kaylani et al., "Neurohemodynamic Correlates of 'OM' Chanting: A Pilot Functional Magnetic Resonance Imaging Study," *International Journal of Yoga*, 2011, available online at http://www.ijoy.org.in/article.asp?issn=0973-6131;year=2011 ;volume=4;issue=1;spage=3;epage=6;aulast=Kalyani.

10. Maheshkumar Kuppusamy et al., "Effects of Bhramari Pranayama on Health—A Sys-tematic Review," *Journal of Traditional and Complementary Medicine*, 2017, available online at https://www.ncbi.nlm.nih.gov/pmc/articles/PMC5755957.

11. R. Jerath, J. W. Edry, V. A. Barnes, and V. Jerath, "Physiology of Long Pranayamic Breathing: Neural Respiratory Elements May Provide a Mechanism That Explains How Slow Deep Breathing Shifts the Autonomic Nervous System," *Medical Hypotheses*, 2006.

12. Xiao Ma et al., "The Effect of Diaphragmatic Breathing on Attention, Negative Affect and Stress in Healthy Adults," *Frontiers in Psychology*, 2017, available online at https:// www.ncbi.nlm.nih.gov/pmc/articles/PMC5455070/.

13. Christopher Bergland, "Why Do the Songs from Your Past Evoke Such Vivid Mem-ories?," *Psychology Today*, December 2013, available online at https://www.psycholo gytoday.com/us/blog/the-athletes-way/201312/why-do-the-songs-your-past-evoke -such-vivid-memories.

14. Viktor Müller and Ulman Lindenberger, "Cardiac and Respiratory Patterns Synchron-ize between Persons during Choir Singing," PLoS One, September 2011, available online at https://journals.plos.org/plosone/article?id=10.1371/journal.pone.0024893.

15. Tom Shakespeare and Alice Whieldon, "Sing Your Heart Out: Community Singing as Part of Mental Health Recovery," *Medical Humanities*, December 2017, available online at https://mh.bmj.com/content/44/3/153.

16. Ilene A. Serlin, "Dancing Away Dementia," *Psychology Today*, November 2013, avail-able online at https://www.psychologytoday.com/us/blog/make-your-life-blessing /201311/dancing-away-dementia.

17. Richard Powers, "Use It or Lose It: Dancing Makes You Smarter, Longer," Stanford Dance, available online at https://socialdance.stanford.edu/syllabi/smarter.htm.

18. H. Steinberg, "Exercise Enhances Creativity Independently of Mood," *British Journal of Sports Medicine*, 1997, available online at https://bjsm.bmj.com/content/bjsports/31/3/240 .full.pdf.

19. K. R. Norman (translator), *The Rhinoceros Horn and Other Early Buddhist Poems* (Sutta-Nipata) (Melksham: Pali Text Society, 1984).

20. Thich Nhat Hanh, *Silence* (New York: HarperOne, 2015), 7.

21. Adam Hadhazy, "Why Does the Sound of Water Help You Sleep?," Live Science, January 2016, https://www.livescience.com/53403-why-sound-of-water-helps-you-sleep.html.

Chapter 17: Out of Touch

1. T. Field et al., "Preterm Infant Massage Therapy Research: A Review," *Infant Behavioral Development*, April 2011, available online at https://www.ncbi.nlm.nih.gov/pmc/articles/PMC2844909/.

2. A. Montagu, *Touching; The Human Significance of the Skin*, Third Edition (New York: Harper & Row Publishers, 1986).

3. Daniel Goleman, "The Experience of Touch: Research Points to a Critical Role," *New York Times*, February 1998, available online at https://www.nytimes.com/1988/02/02/science/the-experience-of-touch-research-points-to-a-critical-role.html.

4. Matthew J. Hertenstein et al., "The Communication of Emotion via Touch," *Emotion*, August 2009, available online at https://www.ncbi.nlm.nih.gov/pubmed/19653781.

5. Valeria Gazzola, "Primary Somatosensory Cortex Discriminates Affective Significance in Social Touch," *Proceedings of the National Academy of Sciences*, June 2012, available online at https://www.ncbi.nlm.nih.gov/pmc/articles/PMC3382530/.

6. Michael Kraus and Dacher Keltner, "Tactile Communication, Cooperation, and Performance: An Ethological Study of the NBA," *Emotion*, October 2010, available online at https://www.researchgate.net/publication/47642304_Tactile_Communication_Cooperation_and_Performance_An_Ethological_Study_of_the_NBA.

7. E. Sommers et al., "Providers of Complementary and Alternative Health Services in Boston Respond to September 11," *American Journal of Public Health*, 2002, available online at https://www.ncbi.nlm.nih.gov/pmc/articles/PMC1447287/.

8. Ian McCafferty, "In Safe Hands: Massage & PTSD," May 2016, *Massage Therapy Journal*, available online at https://www.amtamassage.org/articles/3/MTJ/detail/3484/in-safe-hands-massage-ptsd.

9. B. Ditzen et al., "Effects of Different Kinds of Couple Interaction on Cortisol and Heart Rate Responses to Stress in Women," *Psychoneuroendocrinology*, 2007; "Healing Touch: Hands-on Help for the Heart?," Harvard Health Publishing, March 2014, available online at https://www.health.harvard.edu/newsletter_article/Healing_touch_Hands-on_help_for_the_heart.

Chapter 18: Mindfulness—Tidy Up Your Mind to Stand Taller

1. "Moving through Time: Thinking of the Past or Future Causes Us to Sway Backward or Forward," Science Daily, January 2010, available online at https://www.science daily.com/releases/2010/01/100121135859.htm.

2. Vivian Giang, "The Surprising and Powerful Links Between Posture and Mood," *Fast Company*, January 2015, available online at https://www.fastcompany.com/3041688/the -surprising-and-powerful-links-between-posture-and-mood.

3. Robert M. Pirsig, *Zen and the Art of Motorcycle Maintenance* (New York: HarperTorch, 2006), 303.

4. Lucette Lagnado, "U.S. Probes Use of Antipsychotic Drugs on Children," *Wall Street Journal*, August 2013, available online at https://www.wsj.com/articles/us-probes-use-of -antipsychotic-drugs-on-children-1376275176.

5. "New Survey Reveals Extent, Impact of Information Overload on Workers; From Boston to Beijing, Professionals Feel Overwhelmed, Demoralized," LexisNexis, October 2010, available online at https://www.lexisnexis.com/en-us/about-us/media/press-release.page ?id=128751276114739.

6. Robert Sapolsky, *Why Zebras Don't Get Ulcers*, 3rd Edition (New York: Holt Paperbacks, 2004): 16–17.

7. Daniel J. Siegel, *Aware* (New York: Tarcher Perigree, 2018), 337–338.

8. Kevin Yackle et al., "Breathing Control Center Neurons That Promote Arousal in Mice," *Science*, March 2017, available online at http://science.sciencemag.org/content /355/6332/1411.

9. Alice Park, "This Is the Fastest Way to Calm Down," *Time*, March 2017, available online at http://time.com/4718723/deep-breathing-meditation-calm-anxiety/.

Index